WHEN SITTING
IS NOT RESTING:
SITTING VOLLEYBALL

WHEN SITTING IS NOT RESTING: SITTING VOLLEYBALL

Maciej,

*Thanks for your time
and support,*
Kwok.

Kwok Ng

www.sittingvolleyball.info

authorHOUSE®

AuthorHouse™
1663 Liberty Drive
Bloomington, IN 47403
www.authorhouse.com
Phone: 1-800-839-8640

This edition first published 2012
Copyright © 2012 by Kwok Ng. All rights reserved.

Reprinted December 2012

Published by AuthorHouse   July 27, 2012

ISBN: 978-1-4772-1790-0 (sc)
ISBN: 978-1-4772-1789-4 (hc)
ISBN: 978-1-4772-1791-7 (e)

1 2 3 4 5 6 7 8 9 0

Cover Photo by © Kwok Ng, all other photographs courtesy of Finnish Sports Association of Persons
with Disabilities or private collection of Kwok Ng. Illustrations by © Kwok Ng.

This book is printed on acid-free paper.

CONTENTS

Section 1

Section 2

Section 3

Development in Sitting Volleyball............................. 117

ILLUSTRATIONS

PREFACE

William Morgan has been attributed with inventing the game of Mintonette in 1895, as he created an alternative to basketball. It was later renamed as volleyball. With the help of American troops moving across the world during major international conflicts, the game spread fast throughout Europe and later to the Rest of the World. During the 2012 World Congress of the International Volleyball Federation (FIVB), there were 220 nations as members of the FIVB. This spread of the sport of volleyball has reached out to more nations than the United Nations and the International Olympic Committee. Under a closer inspection of the spread of volleyball, there is a realisation that sport and peace go hand in hand. Since the 1990s, the top two nations in men's Sitting Volleyball have been Iran and Bosnia. Both countries were in major conflicts with their own neighbouring countries during the 1990s, and their countries were victims of many fatalities and casualties. Many men were left without limbs as bombs and mines destructed their homes and conflict zones. In order to continue with everyday life, the survivors had found peace through sporting activities and ultimately found excellence with Sitting Volleyball.

Sitting Volleyball is a modification of the standing game, with the exception of some basic differences. The game is still played with a lot of technical skill and tactical knowledge. It requires quick reactions to play fast moving balls. Volleyball also demands the highest level of team dynamics. With many players covering a small amount of court space, teams have up to three touches to execute an attack shot. This type of essential passing is a result from strong cohesion. In brief, the main differences in Sitting Volleyball include the following; the net is lower; the court is smaller; while playing the ball, the area of the body between the buttocks and shoulders must be in contact with the floor; following a joust, the point is replayed; and, the service block is permitted. This last rule difference is a tactical one and not always adopted by all teams. This book explores some ways in which Sitting Volleyball tactics can be developed for teams.

In order for a coach to transfer knowledge from the standing game to the sitting game, many coaches are often stranded for ideas on how to coach during the game. Many rely on tactics and systems similar to the standing game. At the highest levels coaches often find that it can lead to some success, while teams without specialised consideration for the game will be disadvantaged. This is the first book if its kind. The main content will provide some tactical strategies to help the coach and players to understand the sitting game as played at the international level. Fundamental considerations of team formation, team systems and general tactics are described in some detail within these chapters. The information provided in this book has come from observing and analysing top international teams. Several observation hours were compiled to make this book. Footage of recent top international matches as well as classic matches dating back to 1995 were watched to produce the important facts used in this book. It is also important to note, that there are more ways of successful strategies that this book has not included. It wasn't because other ways to play are not deemed as effective, it is quite possibly the lack of inclusion is because those team systems had not been observed throughout the matches, that game rules have changed since the availability of game footage was used, or simply there wasn't sufficient room to provide detail in this book.

Unlike standing volleyball, the background of elite Sitting Volleyball players is rather diverse. Currently, this is proving to be of interest. Media reporters are interested by the background of disabled athletes. Sporting governance wants to know what types of athletes are playing their sports. Potential sponsors might be looking for athlete endorsement for their targeted campaigns. These interests lead to some broad questions; what is Sitting Volleyball? What are the differences between volleyball and Sitting Volleyball? How is Sitting Volleyball played? What suggestions are there to play Sitting Volleyball beyond the international game? This book tries to address these questions in three sections.

The first section is divided into three more chapters. Chapter two starts by looking at the history of the sport. Here, rummages of available accounts of historical events are collected as one story. Sitting Volleyball is often looked at as a disability sport. Its history of expansion as a disability sport occurred through international competitions, large and small. In this chapter, there are accounts of major competitions, including the World and Zonal Championships since 1976, the year where Sitting Volleyball was a test event for what is now known as the Paralympics. As Sitting Volleyball matured it went from generic disability sports management to having its own governing body formed.

The World Organisation of Volleyball for the Disabled (WOVD) as an organisation is presented in chapter three. Within this chapter, the most current way (in 2012) that the WOVD operates is printed here. Each department is briefly described. This chapter is not intended to claim that it portrays facts about the organisation. No involvement with the WOVD board of administration took place when writing this chapter. The chapter finishes off on the topical area of disability sport; classification. The area of classification as currently defined for Sitting Volleyball is presented, however, over the coming years, the matter may change, and this is something that all disabilities sports are having to experience.

The last chapter in this section, chapter four, describes the rule differences between sitting and indoor volleyball. The rules of the game can be downloaded from the WOVD website and various other national federation websites; however, this chapter focuses on the experience of the rule changes. Over the years, conversations with international referees and referee observers as well as coaches, players and managers have highlighted the importance of knowing the differences between Sitting Volleyball and other types of volleyball. Such information, may eventually act as a case book on the rules of Sitting Volleyball. In its current form, chapter four is presented through a basic overview of the rule differences, areas that pay particular attention if the spectator is new to the game.

The second typically asked question is of how Sitting Volleyball is played, and is briefly conveyed in section 2. The technical aspects of the game have remained the same since de Haan's book on Sitting Volleyball in 1985. For more information about how to produce technical shots, his book is strongly recommended. Bullet points of technical points can also be found in Vute's book on disabled volleyball. Once players have technical skill competencies, players may need to know effective tactics. Others may experience different ways of playing the game as it depends on their teammates and their opponent's abilities.

A look at service reception systems is presented in chapter 5. Systematic observations of international matches between 1999 and 2008 were used to create the findings published in this book. The observing eye sees only certain things, whereby another eye may see another. In order to provide consistency, the observations came from only one observer during years of data collection focusing on tactical systems. In addition to the coaching philosophies spanning over 10 years, there are instructions for understanding the reception systems in Sitting Volleyball. Receiving the ball is only a component of reception systems, the mechanism to form an attack, and an effective sideout is also considered, and examples of various number of setting systems are introduced. Other than receiving and setting for sideout, another valued component of volleyball is defence. Chapter 6 gives some examples of different ways of defence. Using the same data collection methods as in the previous chapter, there are instructions for understanding better defensive systems. Defensive systems forms fundamental processes to winning volleyball games. The ability to save a point and transition to score will make any team hold an advantage other another.

Section three aims to address the third question; what suggestions are there to play Sitting Volleyball beyond the international game. In order to bring this into perspective a chapter summarising the issues surrounding disability sports is available. As a theoretical chapter, a further reading list is available at the end of the chapter. Reviews of current literature, attendance of academic conferences, and conversations with specialists in Physical Education formed the basis for this chapter. It has not been possible to include every angle as the realm of disability sport is vast. Thoughts about certain papers that relate to Sitting Volleyball outside the international game context were considered most relevant.

In the last chapter, the focus on youth sports is presented through studies on training coaches and teachers. A youth competition model is presented in the form of mini-volley and advice on the development stages of youth in relation to Sitting Volleyball is also presented. Although these suggestions are not set in stone by any authority, the ideas have been tested with a small group of students at various stages of development, compiled with literature on pedagogy, psychology of human development, motor testing on children with disabilities, and interviews of experts in coaching youth and volleyball.

Background for the book

It seems very difficult for school children to say the name 'Mr Ng' in English. As such, my aspirations of being a physical education teacher went out the window quite early on in life. However, in order to continue to educate in sports, I looked at the, then vocational subject, of coaching. As a late teenager, I got my first coaching qualification in the sport of Lacrosse. Quite a minority sport around the world, and coaching opportunities were limited. Further coaching qualifications were pursued in a variety of sports. The opportunities to put theory into practice were essential. People wanted experience before gaining a contract. Unlike a teaching degree, whereby trainees learn by teaching, coach qualifications haven't been as structured and opportunities were self-initiated.

I started volunteering at a local club for people with disabilities, coaching a multiple array of sports, for people with various disabilities. Weekly sessions of archery, boccia, bowls, and curling were their favourite activities. Working with multiple disabilities gave me the insight to run inclusive activities. I started to build up a bank of knowledge and became known throughout certain communities that my specialism was in volleyball. Following this, a request came to help and provide volleyball sessions in schools.

After running some successful PE lessons to a special needs school, and using Sitting Volleyball as the focus activity, the teacher asked me, "Is there a book or something where I can get some materials for teaching this game?" I was hesitant to answer, as I was unaware of any such book. After a long pause and a look of worry, the teacher, went on to say, "This lesson was really useful, why don't you make a book on this"? This is the result from such a request. It has taken five years and evolved quite a lot from the origins. During this time, the shift away from special needs to top level international and club Sitting Volleyball formed part of the research process. In addition to acquiring specialist knowledge in adapted physical activities, inclusion sports, practical sessions to test theories, this book contains the first set of results from the accumulated research. Despite the experience of working with national teams and attending coaching seminars, there still alluded an available book that would be helpful for coaches and top sport in Sitting Volleyball. As a self-financed book, it is my hope that this book informs and educates people about the game of Sitting Volleyball.

Beyond the book

One of the issues about books on sports, are the changes that occur over time can often make events outdated. However, the core content of the book should remain relevant for several years to come. For example, the chapter on the history of the game is never ending as history is made every day. It is intended that major competition results that occur after the publication of the book cannot appear in print, but will become available on the website (www.sittingvolleyball.info). Over the years, the rules of the game have changed the way teams play Sitting Volleyball. When major rules changes are introduced, features that eliminate or create new strategies will need to be considered in newer editions. Further additions can provide room for discussions between those involved in the sport.

Another area that should be noted is the use terminology when referring to disability and people. The Publication Manual of the American Psychology Association's 6th Edition states 'person with disability' should be used. However, in the majority of circumstances the term 'disabled person/ athlete/player/child' is used throughout the book. These words are used to describe physical, psychological, mental disabilities and/or impairments which may be offensive or discriminatory reflects the English language, and therefore, is not intended to be offensive or discriminatory to individuals.

To explain this further, I present arguments for alternative and non-offensive ways of writing 'disabled person'. The 'chunking' of these words as 'disabled person' should not in any way intend to demean or offend any person to which this literature relates. Many British authors have contested that the use of political correctness, the use of the person first (such as 'person with a disability), rather than the disability first (such as 'disabled person') is often justified in reference to the way language is portrayed. An example of such a sentence; "training with children with disabilities", rather than; "training with disabled children". The difficulty to follow such prose can detract the reader from the meaning of the text as the sentences become hard to read when using person first statements. The fact that the approach to sports were previously based on institutions for the non-disabled, or there are many references to existing literature make strong casing points in disability studies to continue to use disability first statements. These all provide a rational approach to the manner of social science descriptions.

Furthermore, throughout the world and within the majority of the Sitting Volleyball community, the word 'disabled' is used, as is 'able-bodied'. The highest competition for Sitting Volleyball insists on classified athletes with disabilities, whereby their bodies not fully able. It is not surprising that the athletes themselves refer to people without disabilities as 'able-bodied'. Therefore to simplify the text, the phrase 'non-disabled' is often seen, as oppose to 'people without disabilities', as well as the terms 'disabled person' and 'people with disabilities' can also be found. In this book, there are stylistic issues here in the English used, and it is not intended to be offensive or discriminatory.

Unfortunately, it is very hard to support the American Psychology Association's 6th Edition manual's suggestions of using 'persons with a disability' in this text, as it also refers to a group of individuals having a singular disability. Despite 'disability' being a countable and uncountable noun, using the article 'a' in front, surely means there is only one disability. A person with only one disability can be seen as a medical problem and that is not the current way of interpreting disabilities based on a social way. More about terminology and models of disability is presented in chapter 7.

Acknowledgements

There are many works that deserve mentioning. Understanding the work of other credible academics should not go unnoticed. Some secondary source materials used in these chapters have helped form the philosophy behind this book. A lot of text relating to my earlier studies on adapted physical activity, teacher training, coach evaluations, and volleyball knowledge have been used. It is not easy to list only a few scholarly and application texts that have helped with this book, and therefore a full reference list has not been included. Jouke De Haan's book, titled, 'Sitting Volleyball', and Rajko Vute's "Teaching And Coaching Volleyball For The Disabled" manual are an exception, not because they are the only available text books principally on Sitting Volleyball, the authors have spent the time with me in bringing ideas to the table for this book. Their inspiration to contribute to people interested in Sitting Volleyball is phenomenal, and I could only dream to reach their accolades one day in the future.

This book is not intended to claim that events portrayed in Section 1 are proven historical facts on any organisational, national, or international level. The five years of work that culminated to this book would not have been possible without the support of the Sitting Volleyball community, the academic advisors, and friends, in particular Dixie Brambles. A special mention to Joze Banfi for officially introducing the sport to me. I spent four years in Finland writing this book with the help of the Finnish Sitting Volleyball representatives and their ability to work with me on this is most appreciated. I recognise the great tolerance and support from my family and I would like to thank them and my loved ones for this.

Kwok Ng
May 2012

SECTION 1
Sitting Volleyball – the Sport

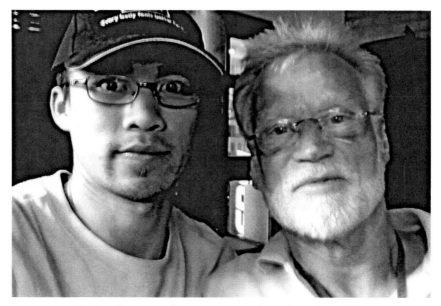

© Kwok Ng with Pieter Joon, founder of WOVD

1 INTRODUCTION

Two teams approach the centre of the court as the announcer names the teams. There is stillness among the crowd. It was time to play the national anthems. The national anthem that was played first was the Star Spangled Banner, the American anthem. What followed was the new anthem of Iraq - Mawtini. In a neutral venue there were Americans and Iraqis. It was a sight that is not seen every day.

During the summer of 2006, the World Championships of Volleyball for the Disabled took place, in Roermond, Netherlands. Both USA and Iraq played against each other for 9th/10th place. The game had significance importance, and it wasn't just for the 9th place result. It could be noted that at that time, the trial following the USA's capture of the Iraq's leader was nearing completion in its second year and a verdict from the court. Troops from the USA Army had lost a limb or two through their service in Iraq featured in the American team. Players in the Iraqi team had friends and families affected by the recent conflict. In some people's eyes, deep wounds from the war may have emotions that would engage more strife between personnel than any other match throughout the tournament. However, it wasn't the time where two groups fought in vain against each other.

There were supposed to be tensions between the two countries however, on the sports field a different reality existed. There was huge emphasis on peace and friendship among this sporting community. A contest was of skills, gamesmanship, talent, team work, and ball skills, not of weapons, warfare, and alliances. Players on the field seem to forget the recent events and concentrated on the match. Ball after ball, until a team won three sets, the players continued on. On this occasion, the American team were victorious. After the game, teams met at the middle of the court, shook hands, some seen to give hugs to each other. The victims of war were brought together through peace and sport. The sport that allowed them this, was Sitting Volleyball.

Sitting Volleyball has an uncanny knack of bringing peace and sport together. The terrorist bombings in London on the 7th July 2005 blew away the limbs of people and lives of others. One survivor from the bombings now plays Sitting Volleyball for her national team. She was later awarded the title of the most inspirational woman in sport for 2012. Also, in the same team, is a former soldier that served in Iraq, when in 2006 she was left paralyzed. As Sitting Volleyball is a new sport in Great Britain, the recruitment of players was direct and there lies strong links between people who were in the services and sport.

From a country of novice players to former world champions, Sitting Volleyball is hugely successful and popular in Bosnia and Herzegovina. It is a country that was torn apart in the Yugoslavian break up during the 1990s. Reports of players that have found solitude from the sport after the civil war are now playing Sitting Volleyball. Players from the Bosnian team went from rehabilitation through to serious competitive training. The results only got better to when they reached the top of the world in 2004 and became household names in the country. Players that were once on the brink of death, consider them to be lucky to be alive. They embrace the sport of Sitting Volleyball and demonstrate peace and friendship through encounters on and off the court.

Sitting Volleyball hasn't been recognised as a means of dealing with post-traumatic stress syndrome, but it might as well, given the number of positive cases that athletes have been through. Many elite athletes found themselves referred by professionals to participate in sport following a traumatic event. But the attribution of Sitting Volleyball as the first solution would be rare. In both modern medicine and homoeopathy, if the sport was solely seen as a means of dealing with post-traumatic stress syndrome, it will probably have to be the sole purpose of it. However, Sitting Volleyball isn't just a cure for dealing with traumatic life events. It is much more. It is a type of volleyball that can be played by virtually all people. In this sense, it is the inclusive version of volleyball.

People that have previously played volleyball may find Sitting Volleyball to be a practical way of exercising, competing and practicing unique skills related to volleyball throughout their lifespan. In many ways, even at the elite level, the average player in Sitting Volleyball is slightly older than the average volleyball player. When landing from jumping the impact and sore joints built over time may restrict the ability to play volleyball in later years. In order to continue practicing the skills learnt from volleyball, Sitting Volleyball acts as a solution to overcome niggling pains. The energy exerted to jump high from indoor volleyball requires a combination of properly attuned trained muscles, energy systems, and abilities to cope with psychological variables. The use of fast twitch muscles used in jumping may deplete over time, and to eliminate being outplayed by younger, stronger athletes who have the capacity to jump, Sitting Volleyball is a game that produces fairness amongst players.

Playing volleyball requires regular practice and contact with the ball. When players experiences some sort of injury, Sitting Volleyball can be a good source of rehabilitation as it caters for the need to practice ball contact and team practices without the risk of making the injury worse. In such cases, Sitting Volleyball can act as a temporary way of practice and contact with the ball. The game conditions players with fast

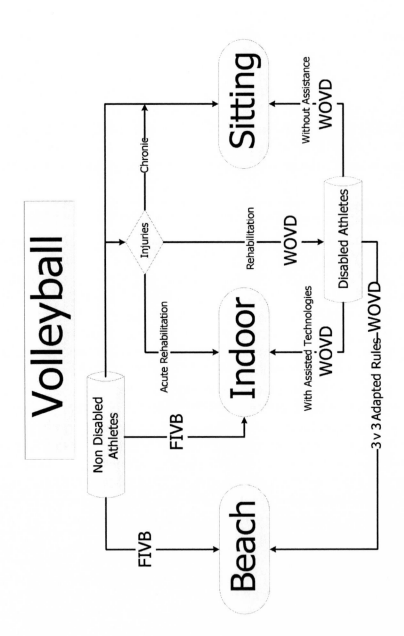

1.Volleyball Sports Participation

reactions and ball control over small distances. As a new challenge to volleyball players, it can be motivating for players to play Sitting Volleyball. No disability, injury or special reason is needed to join in. Therefore, Sitting Volleyball can be regarded as the inclusive version of volleyball. The representation of the player participation of volleyball appears in figure 1.

1.1 **Volleyball**

Volleyball as a sport has grown in every continent, and is recognised in 220 countries. 220 nations in one organisation have made the FIVB the largest sporting body on the planet. With a wide variety of cultures and people, it already makes volleyball a diverse sport. It is played across the globe by professional athletes, amateur players, recreational hobbyists, as well as youth in schools, mums sports clubs, family and friends practicing on the street, playgrounds, grass, beach, even, classrooms while sitting down. The diverse nature of the sport has made the sport successful, and also its weakness. For example, the way the game is played on sand has been so well refined in clear cut ways, that the official beach volleyball game to have its own set of rules. Such differences to the average person who wants to play volleyball needs to be acknowledged in order for them to play a fair game while experiencing the fitness and fun gained through playing beach volleyball. If there are 3 people who turn up on the sand and play as one team, which rules should be kept from the indoor game?, and which rules from the beach game should apply? Who decides? Such difficult decisions amongst friends can typically be a reason for not playing the sport. In other words, volleyball requires some level of organisation before it can be played. Although minor organisational issues, the extra work load for teachers in schools has also seen a reduction in the amount of time to teach volleyball. In chapter 8, there is a section on small-sided game management for Sitting Volleyball.

Although there can often be some difficulties for a group of friends to play volleyball, the group also has the luxury of modifying the rules, number of people, net height and court size based on the number of people who play. With this in mind, similar games that resemble volleyball were known to have been played over 500 years ago on the British Isles. The modern game as we know is flexible in nature. This is a major strength in the development of the game. This has resulted in various forms of the game have been played for people throughout their lifespan. There is mini-volleyball for young children, 9-a-side volleyball leagues for house wife mothers, 12-a-side volleyball for densely populated cities, modified seniors volleyball with lighter balls and lower nets. A lot of these modifications are established ways of playing the game and regular competitions take place using these game versions.

The diverse nature of volleyball is also suitable for people with disabilities too. Depending upon the severity of disability, there are different recognised versions of volleyball; Sitting Volleyball and standing volleyball. Both versions of the sport are recognised internationally and are official sports of the World Organisation of Volleyball for the Disabled (WOVD). Both versions attempt to use as similar rules to the indoor game as possible, with only modifications that allow for fair play and without the scope of abilities due to the athlete's disabilities. For example, in Sitting Volleyball, the game permits the service block, a rule that was taken out of the indoor game in the 1960s. The net height and court size is also modified which keeps the amount of movement, reaction time and space used per person playing the game at a fast pace. The game is just as exciting as all other types of volleyball. While in standing volleyball, only classification rules applies in addition to the FIVB rules.

Even though the game of Sitting Volleyball is similar to the standing game, the way to play it is fundamentally different. As such, it is very surprising to find that there is only one book solely on the sport of Sitting Volleyball by Jouke de Haan. Despite international competition started over 50 years ago, participation in over 50 countries, there is a real need to have some concrete resources that support the development of the sport. There have been the occasional mentions in disability sports text books, and an introductory foundational coaching course manual since de Haan's book was published in 1985, but a modern book is lacking. Since 1985, the game has evolved with the major rule changing the way points are scored. Prior to 2000, volleyball was played using a point-on-serve system. Teams could only score when they served (had the ball) and won that rally. To stop the opponent from scoring, the receiving team needed to side-out and obtain possession of the ball. Now, the game is played under a rally point system, whereby every point counts.

The introduction of the libero was also another fundamental change in team dynamics. A specialist player in the back row gave the opportunity for defensive specialisms and recovery for front row players without taking an official substitution. Another notable change is based on the standards and level of ball handling. In addition to the different look and texture of balls played, from white leather coated balls to multi-coloured panelled balls, playing the first touch had been relaxed to allow flowing rallies. These, and other changes over time, have made slow progressions to the way the game is played today, however a book on modern ideas is, until this book, not been available. Although technical aspects of the games have changed only slightly, de Haan's book still provides excellent reading for Sitting Volleyball techniques, therefore this book looks at some of the typical formations used in Sitting Volleyball so it is less confusing to play, watch and understand.

1.2 Elite Sport in Sitting Volleyball

As a Paralympic event, there are regular major international championships between countries in different parts of the world. In the two year gap between the summer games, the WOVD hosts the world championships, and the winner of this tournament automatically qualifies for the next summer Paralympics. It was in the late 1970s where the International Sports Organisation for the Disabled (ISOD) decided to provide governance to the sports so they would be able to develop their competitions to a more localised audience. The role of the WOVD is the sole communicator with ISOD (now IPC) regarding the Paralympics. The WOVD's infrastructure consists of several regional zones and departments. These regions are based on geography and consists of the European Zone, the America's zone, the African Zone and the Asian Oceanic Zone. Collectively they complete the entire world. Each zone holds zonal tournaments as a qualification process for the Paralympics and the Paralympics comprises 8 teams (10 teams in the men's tournament was introduced for 2012) consisting the top three teams from the world championships, the winner of each of the four zones, and the host nation. For the men's tournament, a separate sub-Saharan zone qualification was a result of a bipartite commission decision for the allocation of the extra places and the top ranked team from the Intercontinental cup makes up the last spot.

The background of players that play Sitting Volleyball is vast. The diverse element makes the game accessible to many people. The majority of top level players that come from post-war countries appear to have high numbers of amputees. In places where there is a high prevalence of diseases such as poliomyelitis, a good proportional of players field their international teams. In Western European countries, more degenerative conditions such as joint fusions are found among players. As such, around the globe, there are groups of disabilities that can find Sitting Volleyball to be a suitable and successful sport to play.

All international athletes must be classified. This classification passport is valid for four years and if the athlete continues to play after the four years are up, they must be re-examined even if they have a very clear and visible disability. The procedures ensure athletes do not cheat. The classification process comprises of, as stipulated by the IPC, three elements; physical examination, motor examination and an observation. It has two purposes; disability eligibility and whom it'll be fair to compete against. The physical examination checks for functionality of the limbs. Furthermore, the motor examination tests the disability with their ability. For some athletes whose disability is not so visible, this kind of test can almost eliminate any signs of cheating created by the athlete during the examination. If the classifiers are still uncertain about how to classify the athlete, they will observe athletes playing the game, to see the overall impact of the injury on the athlete's level of functionality. More information about the levels of classification and the process is in chapter 2.

The term youth Sitting Volleyball, may not appear to be what most of the sporting world would consider to be youth. In some zones, youth tournaments include athletes under 23, while in other zones the age for a junior is also under 23. The age is considered to be quite high in comparison to many other sports for juniors and youth, it could be argued that these athletes are actually fully grown adults and should be playing at senior level Sitting Volleyball. However, the average age of senior national team players tends to be higher than in other sports, and these age group players have greater possibilities to play elite sport hence the younger age group is also older than in other sports. During 2012, the average age of teams competing at the Paralympics was 33 years old for women. While the oldest female player was 55, the youngster player was 14 years old, there are large differences in physical, mental, biological, and volleyball age among those players. In the men's tournament, the average age was slightly lower than with women, at 32 years old, and the oldest athlete was 51 years old and the youngest was 18. Both players were from the same team.

The world junior championships started in 2005 and are held every two years. There are still few nations that enter teams in the national junior championships, and all these teams are men's team. Some zonal championships will permit female players to also play if they desire as long as they fit with the age and classification requirements. This allowance has been accepted because the lack of youth female players around the world to constitute a youth girls or junior women's tournament. Partly the problems of this is the same around most disability sports, as the majority of players acquire disabilities later on in life, while another problem is the provision of sports for disabled youth is often lacking sufficient support.

1.3 Developments in Sitting Volleyball

In every zonal committee of the WOVD there is a development department. By working with the research department, reports from the athletes, coaches and management can identify ways to help develop the sport. An example of what a department does, is to examine the effects of rule changes on the game. Although there have been active investigations to make significant changes in net height, court size and player positions, no significant changes have been accepted, which could indicate the game was thoroughly planned at its inception. Rule differences between the standing and sitting game are publicly available on the WOVD website and publications and can be read in more detail in chapter 4.

Further investigations looked into the values arisen from the game through research and advocacy in developing countries. Vute, conducted a study using the Participation Motivation Inventory on elite Sitting Volleyball athletes at the 1999 European championships. His research reported differences between men's and women motivational factors. Men preferred to play the sport for social interaction, and women tend to play for friendship and personal strength. Another study by adapted physical activity specialist investigated the reasons for participation from players just in the Balkan area. Socialization was very important for the players (mainly men) and participating for rehabilitation scored the lowest.

More recently, health survey data using the Short Form (36) Health Survey version 2 (SF-36v2), on elite Sitting Volleyball players was conducted throughout 2008 by Mustafins. The SF-36v2 is the 2nd version of an international survey with reports of over 140 translations that measures self-reported functional health and well-being in 8 health domains; physical functioning; role-physical; bodily pain; general health; vitality; social functioning; role-emotional; and, mental health. Combining domains can be seen to summaries physical health as well as mental health. After looking at the results of the study, it appears that Sitting Volleyball players have better overall health when compared with other people who have just lost their limbs. The athletes felt greater vitality, which could be a result of being physical active. However, the mental health components scored lower than the norms set by US populations, which could suggest further psychological care is required for the athletes. A similar study conducted 6 years earlier using only a sample population from Japan suggested that the athletes were dissatisfied with their own physical strength and stamina.

An organisation supported by the United Nations; Right to Play, published some refreshing and opportunistic outcomes from integrating persons with disabilities into society through Sitting Volleyball. The report raises attention to the UN Convention on the Rights of Persons with Disabilities, highlighting the acceptance of adapted sports as an acceptable medium that facilitates integration solutions in sports for the disabled. It further highlights an example of Cambodia, a nation where athletes were fear driven by stigma, raised from their own disability and those people who see Sitting Volleyball for the first time are often struck by how a simple change — from standing to sitting — can make a challenging sport accessible to players with limb loss or paralysis, as an even playing field for all athletes regardless of disability.

Although Sitting Volleyball players have some types of disabilities, when they participate in sport, they have as much risk of injury as other people taking part in sport. In training and competition avoiding injuries is important. Following a ten year follow up study of players' injuries, the types of overuse injuries were identified as lower back pain (41%), shoulder pains (18%) and sprains of wrist and fingers

(10%). Coaches and players can find this long term data useful when planning training programs.

Prior to the 2004 Paralympic Games, biomechanical analysis tried to produce a battery test for Sitting Volleyball athletes. For their results to have a greater significance, more Sitting Volleyball athletes using these tests would help define the physiological requirements of a top Sitting Volleyball athlete.

In terms of winning matches, volleyball is a very tactical game. Some unpublished research has been presented by the Finnish Research Institute for Olympic Sports (KIHU), which identified the most important phases in the game. This was the service reception in the women's game and in the men's game, the block proving vital in a teams' success. These results could be attributed to the ability of the player to move.

Studies examining the efficiency of different types of movements in women's Sitting Volleyball showed that players had no distinct advantage in moving forwards, backwards, or sideward, depending on their hand/wrist positioning. There was some evidence to suggest that women were efficient with their movement depending on the way of movement was initiated.

1.4 Future Research in Sitting Volleyball

In terms of research, Sitting Volleyball is very much in its infancy. More physiological studies need to take place and this will help provide a better understanding and profile of Sitting Volleyball athletes. Are athletes with amputees having a far superior advantage over non amputee athletes? What are the advantages and disadvantages of each type? What methods are best used to test the levels of the different athletes of different abilities? How would specific training for successful test results affect the overall performance outcomes?

More biomechanical based studies are taking place that can advise the IPC for future classification rules. Without changes, the classification rules could lead to the demise of the game as there are fewer athletes currently 'suitable' to play the game than 20 years ago. This is not only war related disabilities, but also the level of improvement in prenatal care, better health care systems for early diagnosis of treatable acquiring disabilities, and a greater rise in the levels of obesity. In terms of how it is observed in sedentary behaviours, even playing the sport in between sedentary and moderate sedentary levels of activity can help to improve the health of individuals.

There is the hope that one day the WOVD and the FIVB will be able to form a single organisation, similar to International Tennis Federation. The last chapter of this book will demonstrate some ways which could help the FIVB understand the versatility of Sitting Volleyball as way for grassroots volleyball. Another concern is the creation and validation of an effective tool that can be universally applied for social inclusion through physical activities.

In summary, Sitting Volleyball has been seen as a means of providing peace in sport among people who live through trauma. It is also a sport that athletes value strongly as friendship and social interaction. Perhaps it can be used as a series of treatments akin to anti-depression drugs. It can also be played by volleyball athletes as an alternative exercise. Furthermore, it can be taught as a stepping stone towards volleyball. This book is broken down into several sections. The first section introduces the game, by illustrating the history, organisational structure, and game rules. The second section is a guide for playing systems including, receive offensive, and defensive offensive systems. The third section summaries the game of Sitting Volleyball for sports for all models.

2 ORGANISATIONAL STRUCTURE

Volleyball's top down structure consists of the International Federation, the Continental Zones, followed by Regions and lastly National Federations. The same basic structure that is within the International Volleyball Federation (FIVB) appears in the World Organisation of Volleyball for the Disabled (WOVD). However, the historical evolution of the FIVB formed and how the WOVD was formed have two very different histories. Since this book focuses more on Sitting Volleyball than that of able-bodied volleyball, space limits a thorough description of the evolution of the FIVB. However, it is worth noting that in 2012, 65 years after its formation, the FIVB consists of 220 affiliated member nations. This number exceeds the number of countries that are part of the United Nations. There are also fewer nations that are members of the International Olympic Committee. The number of member nations in the FIVB even surpasses the membership of the body that looks after, what could be said as, the most popular sport in the world; Football! The way the FIVB promoted itself to far reaching countries is astonishing and that is another story in itself. These are important facts, facts that might be significant and could be taken into consideration when reading about the history of Paralympic Games and what was recommended to the WOVD by the IPC when standing volleyball was dropped from their summer games programme.

The WOVD was part of an evolutionary process that virtually all disability sports had to endure. As a sporting body, it has influences from volleyball federations, military organisations, and disability sports associations. The WOVD is currently a voluntary run non-profit making organisation, with basic principles and expanding strategic goals. As such, there is much room for growth and development, within the organisation and its partners.

To this day, Sitting Volleyball lacks formal recognition by the FIVB. Since the turn of the century, several National Federations of volleyball have incorporated Sitting Volleyball as part of their sporting infrastructure along with indoor standing and beach volleyball. As this movement amongst federations gets stronger, the bottom-up approach by the federations and zones can change the way the FIVB operates. It is hoped that special task forces will help the FIVB to accept disability volleyball and commence an official cooperation programme between the two governing bodies.

2.1 WOVD Structure

The WOVD is the international federation for all volleyball games for people with physical disabilities. They consult players, coaches, officials of the game, and other stakeholders, thus giving them authority to communicate directly with the IPC. In doing so, the WOVD operates following a bottom-up approach. Member states represent the continental zones, and the four zones are the driving force behind the success of the WOVD. Although Sitting Volleyball is just one discipline of volleyball and it has the highest profile in terms of inter-national competition, all other disabled volleyball disciplines have equal status within the organisation. Therefore the WOVD takes care of indoor standing and sitting, and beach standing and sitting. The beach games are still developing and are part of an evolving process. As the beach games start to grow in familiarity, so is the potential for growth and perhaps inclusion as another event at the Paralympics.

There is a board of administration that represents the WOVD at the general assembly. The board members are volunteers, and the organisation is non-profit, while maintaining the highest level of professionalism to improve both the internal and external image. No one individual or a group of individuals are able to manage the complex issues faced by the WOVD in current and future events on their own. The WOVD acts as a uniform group that aims to cover the entire interest of the WOVD community.

A lot of the disabled volleyball community activity is operated on a zonal level and frequently at a national level. The WOVD can assist with providing information and best practices are exchanged. In this way, the WOVD are the sole liaising body for global communications with other international organisations.

2.1.1 **Board of Administration**

The WOVD's organisational structure is currently broken down into the Board of Administration and President, who conducts the General assembly. There is the general management that looks after the daily affairs, such as internal communication, memberships, the finances, and human resources. There are then the Management Committees that work with the President. The standing members of the Board of Administration include Zonal Representatives, Sport Development Department, Development Department, and Marketing Department representatives. Therefore the entire board of administration consists of the following members; President, Sport Director, Development Director, Marketing Director, four zonal presidents, currently European Zone, Africa Zone, Asia Zone, Pan American Zone, and the General Manager, who has no voting rights. A closer look at the structure can be seen in figure 2.

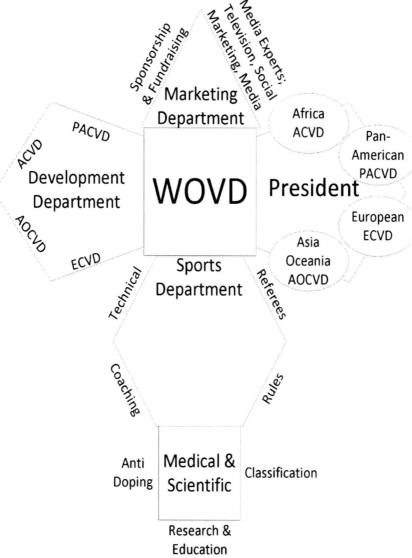

2. Overall Organisation of the WOVD, 2012

The management committee consists of the President, the Sport Director, the General Manager and one zone president, who can act as the vice president. As in many other organisations, the vice president can preside over meetings if the president is otherwise unavailable.

The Sport Director is responsible over a variety of commissions that are related to the sport. These commissions include; Referee commissions, Rules of the Game, Technical Commission, Coaches commission, and the Medical & Scientific commissions, which has three more commissions; Classification, Anti-Doping, and Research & Education. Each commission can work on their own project that coincides with the WOVD strategic plan, a plan that places equal weight towards different types of volleyball for the physically disabled.

The Development Director has fewer commissions to work with, but has still an important role in the development of the WOVD. In order to coordinate the four zones in the WOVD, a chair for the development is needed. Furthermore, a development fund commission is provisioned when there is a need to allocate funds that meet the development criteria.

The Marketing Department operates slightly differently from the development and sport departments. In addition to working with the individual zonal marketing departments that make up a commission, the department consists of a network of experts in television, social marketing, sponsorship, media, and funding.

2.1.2 Sport Department

The Sport department covers the most varied amount of components within the WOVD. In its former guise, it was held as two different departments; sport development, and competition management. The merger of the two have seen how the two previous working departments overlapped with each other and formulated two more commissions that are important to the sport. Previously, the sport development department looked after each of its own goals, commonly; women, youth, education, research, promotion/external communication, and expert platforms of specialities. These goals still play an important role in the way the sport is organised, although some areas have been shifted to the

Marketing department, such as promotion/external communications. Likewise, the Competition Manager, now known as the Sport Director, used to be responsible for the technical committee, referee committee, classification committee, and rules committee. These committees have been turned into commissions and all operate under the sports director leadership in the sport department. In addition to the previous goals and committees, a new commission has been formed. This new commission, namely the coaching commision, plays an important part in the way this disability sport is developed.

The role of the coaching commission is to ensure that a uniform coaching qualification can be recognised internationally. Tutors who deliver coaching courses must be aware of the consistency needed when awarding certification to participants. Since Sitting Volleyball has the highest profile in terms of sport for the physically disabled, it requires special attention in the delivery of a recognised course and certification process. Sitting Volleyball also has a number of differences that need to be observed by coaches that do not simply appear in other volleyball coach training materials. As such, the commission has the intention to investigate in providing a consistent provision for coach training. A key outcome from their work would be to ensure coaches would have had the same amount of time spent on training, and received the same curriculum as other have received from around the world.

Other courses that the WOVD endorse are referee courses and technical courses. The refereeing courses are designed to convert the indoor standing refereeing skills to the game for the disabled. The process of becoming a WOVD referee involves passing the theory and practical examination held at a WOVD course, followed by a series of observations at tournaments. Once referees have gained sufficient experience, they can continue to work with the WOVD as referee observers. Again, they need to attend a course to be officially recognised as a referee observer. The characteristics of the beach game are quite different from the indoor and sitting game. Therefore, another course is designed for beach referees.

Technical courses held by the WOVD mainly consist of a classification course. Classification candidates must meet the minimum requirement, usually holding an equivalent to a doctor or physiotherapist. Once met the criteria, attendance of a short course is needed to provide the theory and practice of classification techniques. Attendance of classification tournaments in both sitting and standing volleyball is necessary before the candidate passes the status as an official classifier. Classification appointments are conducted by the medical and scientific commission, which has three further specific commissions; anti-doping, research and education, and classification. There could also be a further split between the types of classification for the different disciplines of volleyball; standing, sitting, and beach.

2.2 Classification

The purpose of classification is to group together athletes who have the potential for equal movement abilities. Prior to 1992, classification was based mainly by disability group. For the next decade, functional classification was introduced and enhanced. Some combining of classes had to take place to ensure that there were enough athletes to make a competition viable. Currently, there are sport specific classifications and the International Paralympic Committee play a major role in the application of medical support and advice for sport classification systems.

Classifiers are qualified trained personnel with some professional background in movement kinesiology, such as a doctor or physiotherapist. A technical classifier can be a trained person with some experience as a player, coach, or has technical knowledge of the sport. The role of the classifier is made harder because the range of disabilities is enormous; there is a need for a workable number of classes to allow competition to be run, as well as the fact that people can have fluctuating disabilities. The classifier must take only the functional or physical abilities and not their technical skill or success in the sport into consideration.

Classification in Sitting Volleyball is currently based on three tiers. In the most basic form these tiers are defined as; disabled, minimally disabled, and able bodied. As these are the terms used by the athletes, coaches, managers, and classifiers within the sport, any political correctness issues are omitted for the sake of the sport specific classification. Although the United Nations changed its terminology in the 'Rights of the Disabled People' to 'Rights for Persons with disabilities', there are many views that state the reason why the players can play in this sport at classification event, is because they have some type of disability that impedes on their ability to play other forms of volleyball. This notion remains consistent in disability sport literature. Coinciding with the reason for people with disabilities playing disabled sports, the common practice among the disability community in Sitting Volleyball has coined up three short and simple to understand acronyms. In short, players are often referred to as abbreviated terms; D (disabled), MD (minimally disabled), and AB (able bodied).

The process of checking for disability is compulsory for all athletes in sanctioned and official WOVD events. If there is a clear visible disability, that exceeds the minimal disability criteria, then the athlete is given a disability passport to play at the sanctioned competitions. Depending on whether the disability is permanent or is temporary, the permanent passport requires renewal at least once every four years. Athletes that have less severe physical disabilities may be subject to a thorough classification check. The process involves a physical test, perhaps a functional test, and if necessary, an observation. How the classifiers decided upon which level of the classification process goes, depends largely on the type of disability. Volleyball classification is based upon a hybrid model of function and disability type. Very often, the athletes are mainly classed under the 'Amputees and Les Autres' group of disabilities as defined by the International Sports Organisation for the Disabled (ISOD). Other disability types, such as Cerebral Palsy and Wheelchair sports can also be for volleyball athletes. As a result, the hybrid model of classification can be used, whereby function and disability form the criteria for classification. Under the ISOD system for Amputees and Les Autres, the variables examined and criteria is seen in table1;

Table 1. The 1999 Classification of Sitting Volleyball Players for MD

Level of amputation	*Upper limb:* *a) amputation of the first two fingers on two hands;* *b) amputation of seven or more fingers on two hands;* *c) amputation on one hand between the M.P. joint and the wrist;* *Lower limb:* *a) amputation in Lisfranc joint on one foot;* *b) amputation in Chopart joint on one foot.*
Muscle strength	*A minimum decrease in muscle strength of 20 points to include both upper limbs when testing on the 0.5 scale grade system (not counting 1 and 2);* *Each upper limb obtains 70 points, including forearm supination and pronation. The muscle tests on the fingers and thumb being taken into consideration.*
Joint range of movement	*Displasia or luxation of the coxae, Total endoprothesis of knee or hip(s), Very severe circulation defect of lower limb(s), Psuedoarticulation of lower limbs(s), Instability forward/backward of 1.5cms of the knee, Luxation of humeroscapular joint.*
Difference in limb length	*On one upper limb of more than 33%. The shortening must be real or functional in the distance between the acromion and the end of the longest finger as compared to the other limb.*

Observations of new classifications and temporary classified players are a must for all classifiers. In addition to seeing how the athlete performs with their disability, borderline cases between tiers of disability often require a lot of observations before a condition is treated as permanent.

Classifiers are strictly health professionals and provide an evaluation based on their observations and test results. Occasionally, teams may feel that the assessment is incorrect. In this case, there can often be protests against the classification of the athlete. Teams may protest against a lowered classification (e.g. classifying an athlete from D to MD), and other teams can also protest against classification of players in other teams that are higher classifications (e.g. classifying an athlete that was MD to D). Since classifiers cannot discuss any specifics about a player's medical condition or classification assessment with anyone else without breaching ethical practices, teams may find themselves in unfavourable conditions once the competition has begun. The outcomes of classification and protests need to take place well in advance of the important phases of the sanctioned tournaments.

In some cases, teams find that their appeal against a classification unsuccessful. This can often cause line-up changes in the team, sometimes, sending the player back home as they become illegitimate to play. Under the current system, the classification takes place at a time arranged by the tournament organiser, and classifications can remain temporary between sanctioned tournaments. However, during the time between tournaments, players may train to improve their ability to play, and thus find ways to overcome their disability. When the observational tests arise again, the player, who has trained hard since the previous tournament may appear to be stronger, faster and have less disability. Players take time to train and improve in preparation to the major competition, without the certainty they can play at all in a tournament. This can produce a lot of stress and anxiety, factors that can often inhibit their ability to perform. Ultimately, such factors may have an effect on the way the team plays and the result from the game. Furthermore, coaches will have to work with a different set of players with different specialities. This could mean a change in the overall approach, strategy and tactics in the game.

Classification has some of the purist principles designed for disability sports. The purpose is to group people with the same potential for movement together. The way Sitting Volleyball classification has been brought together is from ISOD's amputee and Les Autres systems, which dominated the disability specific criteria for classification. Since the turn of the 21st century, more disability sports recognise the need for sport specific classifications systems. As the sport waits for a new Sitting Volleyball classification system, it might want to also consider the way the process takes places. Classifications might also want to consider the time it takes in relation to the competition before conducting assessments of borderline cases. The process of when and how to classify athletes still remains a large topic for virtually all disability sports; Sitting Volleyball is no different.

3 HISTORY OF SITTING VOLLEYBALL

In 1895, William J Morgan adapted basketball and made a game that was less visible. Later this game was called volleyball. Basketball had only just been adopted among YMCA institutes and it appeared the game that had been played since ancient Greek times, was modernised into the American establishments. Basketball is an invasion game, and in the ruthless age of football, rugby and basketball, a gentler game was necessary. Hence a net game that would separate the teams and reduce the amount of physical contact between players was needed. The troubles it faced were to devise a less physical but recognisable sport and an activity with high demands. While in other invasion games, the ball can be held, and therefore players could catch their breath while holding onto possession of the ball and have the ability to score, games that use a net to separate teams are based on the minimal amount of contact time with the ball or shuttle and that would help them score. Other net games limit the amounts of contacts to a single touch, whereas volleyball, as a team sport supported multiple contacts before the ball went over the net.

The excitement from volleying and rebounding a ball has been popularised throughout the world, among families and top level athletes, and to ensure the game can develop, the international organisation for volleyball (FIVB), was formed in 1947. Forty years after this, the game of beach volleyball that was rooted in Santa Monica, California in the 1920s was later accepted as a sport in the FIVB. Around the same time, the game of Sitting Volleyball was devised and modified to suit players who wanted to play the game without the demands of jumping and landing. In the Netherlands, a game was played by amputees, while in Germany, a similar game called sitzball was played by war veterans. When the two nations came together to play an informal game in 1956, the game of Sitting Volleyball was invented by the Dutch, and later the rules were adopted.

Sitting Volleyball featured as a sport of ISOD in 1976 as a demonstration event. Four years later, disabled volleyball was an officially recognised disability sport led by Pieter Joon from the Netherlands. The WOVD commenced as a standalone sporting body in 1992, following the division of ISOD and the emergence of the International Paralympic Committee.

It may be of interest for the FIVB to recognise volleyball for the disabled. One source of becoming disabled is through chronic injury, and volleyball players' injury prevalence remains high. The FIVB have frequently been seen to turn its head away from disability sports. As the FIVB have looked towards beach volleyball to expand the profile of volleyball around the world, certain zones made their own attempts to put disability sports on their radar by including demonstration events of Sitting Volleyball on the sand. These events were the first time reported by the FIVB media. However, a couple of days later, the pages disappeared from the FIVB website. The reasons for removal remain unknown.

Following to further pressures, the FIVB made one step forward in recognising disability volleyball. During the first FIVB medical congress 2011 in Bled, Slovenia, a keynote speaker on the topic of the Paralympic volleyball athlete was invited, and it was hoped it has paved way for sports medicine interest in Sitting Volleyball athletes. Despite these advances, it still seems to be a long way before the FIVB and the WOVD will cooperate together in volleyball. The past president of the International Paralympic Committee, Robert Steadward had already suggested to the WOVD that volleyball should look towards the International Tennis Federation for the merger of both disability (quad) tennis and non-disabled tennis as a model for inclusion. This announcement came around the time when standing volleyball was removed from the Paralympic programme. With the cooperation between the IPC and the IOC extended further, perhaps there are more opportunities in the future for the WOVD and the FIVB to find ways to cooperate and endorse disability volleyball.

3.1 Sitting Volleyball Competitions

The most prestigious Sitting Volleyball event is the Paralympics. All the major competitions either directly or indirectly give qualification to these summer games. Once every four years, teams fight for the gold medal in the multi-sport competition that is the largest sports competition for people with physical disabilities. The qualification route varies from games to games; however, the most basic way is to gain the berth is through the world championships, which are held every two years between the Paralympics. Zonal competitions can give qualification rights to the world championships if held before that year. Since zonal championships can take place in the year after the world championships, another qualification route is through that tournament too. In some zones, there are ParaPan games, and this also becomes a gateway for qualification.

The following sections provide information about the major international tournaments that go as far back as records tell. Some results still remain missing, although help from various sources around the world, such the Finnish and Japanese Associations as well as the WOVD and ECVD. This is the first time this information is compiled together in English and a summary of the results can be found on the book's website.

3.2 **Previous Competitions**

The first record of international Sitting Volleyball competitions began in 1967, whereby Germany, Netherlands, Sweden and Denmark competed in Flensburg. Prior to this time, the Germans had been used to playing a game called 'Sitzball'. Whereas, the Dutch teams were accustomed to playing a passive form of volleyball played sitting down. During the 1967 tournament, the directors decided to not play the 'sitzball' rules and instead played volleyball sitting down. A year later, a club tournament was organised between teams in Germany (the hosts), Netherlands, and Belgium. Each club had brought their own style to the tournament, whereby the Belgium team had played 'Prellball', the Dutch team played 'Fistball', and the Germans played 'Sitting Volleyball'. The chaos that arose from these early competitions sparked an interest into codifying rules for international competitions.

3.2.1 **1976 – 1984 Variations and Dutch courage**

In the lead up to the 1976 Montreal games, Sitting Volleyball had been played across several countries, and the Stoke Mandeville Games were becoming hugely successful, as was volleyball. With these two events, Sitting Volleyball became a demonstration event with four nations playing the game. However, unlike other demonstration events, whereby the tournament was held at same place as the main games, Sitting Volleyball was demonstrated in Bonn, Germany. Germany won this tournament, with Netherlands second, Finland third and Luxembourg fourth. A lot of change was occurring within the disability sports world. Sir Ludwig Guttmann, the person behind the Stoke Mandeville Games, had wanted to have international sports competition for people with disabilities in the same city as the Olympic Games. Although this vision had been gaining success, the fifth games would run into problems. According to sources, Jean Stone (secretary to the IPC sports council, women in sport committee) suggested

1976-1984

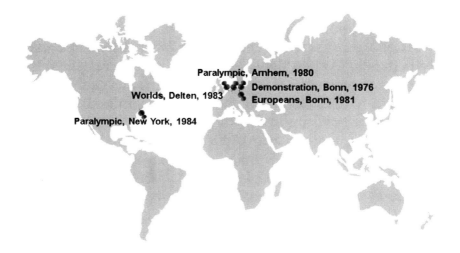

3. Map of competition venues 1976-1984

that the official view of the Soviet Union was that there were 'no disabled people in the Soviet Union'. In order to maintain the momentum achieved by the Paralympic Games, Arhem, in the Netherlands offered and were accepted to host the games. These games would become the turning point in the Paralympics history. As well as including more types of disabilities into the programme, which included the acceptance of both Sitting Volleyball and standing volleyball, it was the first games where the founder, Sir Ludwig Guttmann was unable to attend. He had passed away two months before the opening ceremony, whereby Her Royal Highness Princess Margriet of the Netherlands, declared the 1980 'Olympics for the Disabled' open.

A year later, the first European Sitting Volleyball Championships were held in Bonn, Germany. 10 teams competed and the Netherlands continued to dominate over Germany, who finished second, while Sweden came in third after beating neighbouring Finland in the Bronze medal match. This was the last major competition with the net at

31

1.20m. A change to the net height to 1.15m took place there after and has remained the same ever since. Furthermore, classification of Sitting Volleyball players began using the minimal disability criteria and not the full standing volleyball classification criteria.

In 1983, the first world championships were held in Delten, Netherlands. Despite the title of World Championships, the teams were only from Europe. The Netherlands continued to dominate, with Germany second. However Finland, who had continually ended up in fourth place for the last two major tournaments, managed to capture the bronze medal over neighbouring Sweden. Hungary appeared for the first time with a commendable 7th place finish, ahead of Austria and Denmark. Whereas, in these championships, two nations had ceased to compete; Luxembourg and Belgium, and have since yet to reappear in any future major international competitions.

Since the 1984 Paralympics was divided into two countries London and New York, the Sitting Volleyball tournament was held only in New York. This gave the opportunity for a USA team to appear on the international radar. The Netherlands remain the dominant force in Sitting Volleyball. Once again, the Netherlands beat Germany in the final, however in the Bronze medal match, the rivalry between Sweden and Finland went in favour of the Swedes. Yugoslavia, Norway, USA, and Egypt took up the other places respectively.

3.2.2 1985 – 1992 Iranian Dominance

The 1985 World Championships were held in Kristiansand, Norway. 10 teams entered, and this was the first year where the dominance of the Netherlands had finally been overthrown. A new world champion arrived, and this team was Iran, who fought off Yugoslavia in the finals. The Netherlands ended up with the bronze medal after beating Sweden in the 3rd – 4th place play off. With Germany slipping back into 7th place, Norway increased their position to 5th and Hungary finished also one place better than their debut performance, where

1985-1992

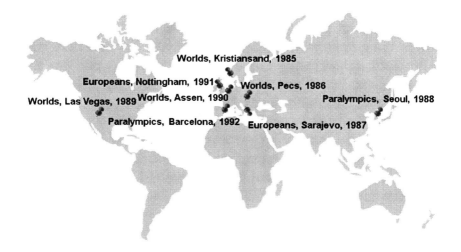

4. Map of competition venues 1985-1992

they ended up in 6th place. Finland had also slipped back to 8th place, while Austria ended up 9th. The Great Britain team debuted at this tournament and finished in last place.

Iran continued as world champion in the following year, as the World Championships took place in Pecs, Hungary. The 1986 Championships were the most successful to date, with a total of 13 teams that participated. Under, what could be called 'home advantage', Hungary lost out to the World Champions, in the Final and claimed a silver medal. The Netherlands claimed 3rd place by beating Yugoslavia and with Sweden with a weakened squad, all other teams up to 7th place picked up one better place than the previous year, as Sweden fell to 8th place. The 1986 tournament saw a return of the USA and GB team, where both teams ended up last, and the Czechoslovakian team competing for their one and only time in major competitions, finishing in 10th place, ahead of Egypt, but after Austria.

The Netherlands managed to reclaim top position after beating hosts, Yugoslavia in the final of the 1987 European

Championships, held in Sarajevo, Yugoslavia. There were again 13 teams in the tournament, three of which came from outside of Europe as they prepared for the following year's major championship. Since the Netherlands had returned to winning forms, the subsequent year was the Paralympic year, where the games were held in Seoul, South Korea. There was a fantastic opportunity for the Netherlands to reclaim the top position, but it wasn't meant to be, as they fell to Iran in the final. This was Iran's first Paralympic gold. Norway played off the bronze medal match with Yugoslavia and was victorious. The remaining positions were filled by, in order; Hungary, Germany, Sweden, South Korea, Egypt, and in last place USA. As hosts, South Korea, finished 8th in a 10 team tournament and their result has, so far, been recorded as the best debut performance by a host nation since the Sitting Volleyball tournament began.

3.2.3 **1993 – 1999 Women Tournaments and unsettled Men in Europe**

1993 would mark a new era in Sitting Volleyball. The European Championships for both men and women were held in Jävenpää, Finland. The tournament was the 5th Men's championships and the first for women. A new European Champion was awarded to Norway, who beat Finland in the Final. In the women's competition, 4 teams competed and the Netherlands edged out Finland 15-12 in the 5th set to clinch the gold medal. Estonia ended up in 3rd place ahead of Latvia.

A year later, the World Championships were also for men and women and it was held in Bottrop, Germany. Iran continued to stamp its authority on the men Sitting Volleyball competition where they beat Norway in the final. The Netherlands beat Finland in the 3rd/4th play-off match. The Netherlands were crowned the first women World Champions as they beat Latvia in the final. Lithuania had to beat Russia to claim 3rd place and Germany took 5th place after beating Ukraine, who finished last in the 6 team tournament.

1993-1999

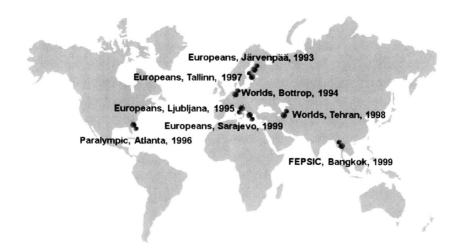

5. Map of competition venues 1993-1999

The following European Championships had different champions. The 1995 tournament in Kamnik, Slovenia, saw Hungary on top, and for the women competition, the Netherlands retained their status as European Champion. A couple of years later, Finland won the European Championship held in Tallinn, Estonia, while Latvia won their first European Championship in the women's competition.

Between these years, teams that had qualified, went to Atlanta, USA for the Paralympic Games. Again, Iran took the gold after beating the 1994 World Championships Silver Medallists, Norway. Finland was able to overcome the Netherlands in the 3rd-4th play-off game to take the Bronze medal. The 1996 games were the first time records show Argentina had competed in a major international competition, and they finished in last position. It is also the last time they have competed.

Following the success of Finland in the European Championships of 1997, it was their turn to fight for the gold medal at the 1998 World Championships against Iran. However, even the Finnish 'sisu' was unable to stand up against the Iranian Sitting Volleyball team. Bosnia and

Herzegovina had come out from the Yugoslavian break up with an abundance of players. They moved up to 3rd place by beating the Netherlands in the play-off game. The women World Championships took place in Germany later that year.

The year before the Sydney Games, the European Championships for men and women were held in Sarajevo, Bosnia and Herzegovina. The rapid pace of Sitting Volleyball development in the former Yugoslavian states brought great success. The game was rapidly becoming a popular sport among the communities. It was a place where socialisation and fitness combined together. A spirit from the aftermath of war was attributed in the way the sport had rapidly developed. Bosnia's neighbour, Slovenia won the women championship as they beat Finland in the final.

It was also the year where teams in Asia competed in the FEPSIC games. Iran beat Japan in the final in Bangkok, Thailand. Iran had already qualified for the Paralympics in Sydney, and a zonal qualifier in Australia was held later in the year, where Japan came out top and Korea also qualified.

3.2.4 2000 – 2002 Rally Point Systems and Bosnia

Outside of volleyball, a lot of controversy took place during the Sydney Paralympics, in particular the issue surrounding the Spanish intellectually disabled basketball team. This led to banning athletes with intellectual disabilities into the Paralympics. It also highlighted the need for the way of classification needs to be reviewed. While this was happening, probably the biggest rule change in the game of volleyball was adopted. In 2000, volleyball would be played based on rally point. The point-on-serve scoring method had ended so that, irrespective of whether the team had served or not, they had a chance to score a point. It was also the last games where standing volleyball was accepted into the Paralympic programme. However, the Sitting Volleyball tournament, with the new way of scoring, was still exciting. In the 12 man tournament, Iran remained dominant, although the young

2000-2002

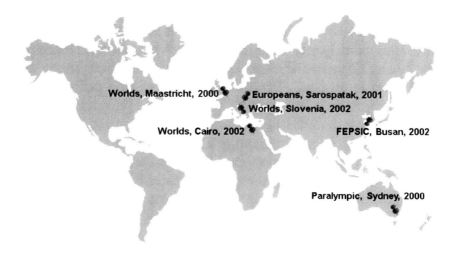

6. Map of competition venues 2000-2002

Bosnian team that began to shine in Europe had just lost out in the Final. Finland took the bronze medal after they beat Egypt. Germany, Netherlands, and Hungary battled out for 5th-7th place. It was the first time that Libya had competed in a major championship and finished in a commendable 8th place a head of Japan, Korea, Australia and Team USA.

Since the women's tournament was not part of the Paralympic programme, there was a separate World Championships for women, held in Maastricht, Netherlands, with the home team taking first place. Finland took silver, and Slovenia won bronze after beating Germany. Japan was the highest ranked team outside of Europe, with a 5th place finish and teams from Mongolia, Ukraine and Iran made up the 8 team tournament.

Bosnia and Herzegovina retained their title of European Champions in 2001, even with the new rules. The European Championships for both men and women were held in Sarospatak, Hungary. The Netherlands continued to dominate women Sitting Volleyball as they also retained the gold medal for the European Championships after beating Slovenia in the final.

In 2002, the world championships were held in two different locations. Men competed in Cario, Egypt, and the women competed in Kamnik, Slovenia. It wasn't the year for Iran, and they could only manage a bronze medal after beating the hosts, Egypt in the 3rd/4th placement match. In an all European team final, Bosnia and Herzegovina pulled off a victory over the best finish a German team had managed to achieve since the 1984 Paralympic Games. Morocco made its debut on the major international competitions circuit and beat USA to finish 9th to avoid last place. There were no signs that the Netherlands would not continue to dominate Sitting Volleyball for women as they beat the hosts Slovenia in the finals. China entered for the first time and finished just outside the medals by losing to Finland in the bronze medal match.

Iran when on to play at the FEPSIC games in Busan, Korea to defend their Asian title, which they duly did by beating Japan once again in the Final. Since there was no women's competition at FEPSIC, the Asia Championships was held in Narita, Japan, where China came out top after beating hosts Japan in the final. Mongolia finished in third place in a 3 team tournament.

3.2.5 2003 – 2007 Global Zonal Games

Up until this point, Europe and Asia were the only continents with a major competition organised by a WOVD zone. Though, the Asia zonal tournaments were still small. This gave European teams a huge advantage over teams outside of Europe, as there were opportunities for high level international competitions. The qualification of teams like Egypt and USA did not come through from zonal qualifiers, whereas, the European teams had to compete in the European Championships and finish well to be given the opportunity to compete in the Paralympics. Since teams had to win the

2003-2007

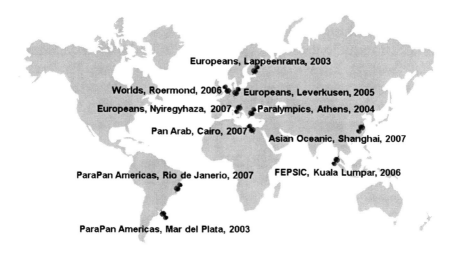

Europeans, Lappeenranta, 2003

Worlds, Roermond, 2006 Europeans, Leverkusen, 2005

Europeans, Nyiregyhaza, 2007 Paralympics, Athens, 2004

Pan Arab, Cairo, 2007

Asian Oceanic, Shanghai, 2007

ParaPan Americas, Rio de Janerio, 2007 FEPSIC, Kuala Lumpar, 2006

ParaPan Americas, Mar del Plata, 2003

7. Map of competition venues 2003-2007

competition to qualify, it systematically increased the level of competition and the professionalism of the sport.

Sitting Volleyball's debut in the America's zonal championships was in Mar del Plata, Argentina, the venue of the 2nd Parapan American Games, 2003. Unlike Europe, the Americas continent holds its own continental multisport competition. The Paralympic sport movement had realised its importance to cooperate with the 13th Pan American Games, Winnipeg, CA in 1999. As negotiations went on, the first Parapan American Games was held in a different city and country. Mexico City became the host city for the first Parapan Games in 1999. As a successful event and under the Paralympic movement, the 2003 and onwards games would be held in the same cities and it was at this event, where Sitting Volleyball had its continental championships. The USA team beat off the Brazilian team in a two horse race. The result was the same for the competition for women teams, whereby the Americas beat Brazil in a two team competition. This gave the US team the right to play in the 2004 Paralympics men competition and the first women Paralympic Sitting Volleyball competition.

Meanwhile in Europe, the European Championships were held in Lappeenranta, Finland. Bosnia continued to demonstrate its striking force on the sitting court as they once again beat Germany in the final. The hosts, Finland took the bronze after beating Russia in the 3rd/4th play-off game. Finland's other bronze medal came in the women's tournament, where the came from behind, 20-24 in the first set, to win the game 3-0, and thus earned a place in Athens. The Netherlands beat Slovenia in the final.

The Athens Games in 2004 saw the inclusion of the women's Sitting Volleyball competition. It was also the first Paralympics since 1976, where volleyball was a single event. Standing volleyball's last appearance was in Sydney as the WOVD failed to meet the newly defined criteria for sport inclusion. The IPC had decided that demonstration sports, with 'demonstration medals' created two classes of athletes, demonstration athletes and full athletes. This did not suit the Paralympic and Olympic model and it was agreed at the beginning of 1997 that sports need to apply 4 years in advance to become included in the Paralympic Programme, and that they needed approval, rather than be tested as a demonstration event. Subsequently, an inclusion criterion was made, which stated that team sports must be practised in 18 countries and three regions. Taking the new ruling into consideration, standing volleyball had failed to meet this criteria for the past five years leading up to the 2000 games. The IPC also became more interested in the Minimal Disability classification of athletes, a classification that was first created for Sitting Volleyball athletes. So, although the standing volleyball competition for men was dropped, a new women's event became available.

There were 8 teams for the men's and 6 teams for the women's tournament in Athens. Bosnia and Herzegovina had been building up their momentum to dominate the Sitting Volleyball world by winning everything they could possibly win after the Sydney Games. The final test came when they played against Iran in the Final for Paralympic Gold. They prevailed and took the gold medal, the first time Iran had not won the gold medal at the Paralympics. The Russian men's team got the last medal, after beating Egypt in the bronze classification game. In the women's tournament, The Netherlands entered the tournament as favourites. Although they were aware of the tough level of competition made available by the European counterparts, the eventual winners, China, had made tremendous progress since the 2002 World Championships. China's MD player did not appear throughout the entire tournament until the final, where they beat the Netherlands 3-1. The only team to have taken a set from China in the entire tournament were the Dutch. The other surprise result came from the USA women's team. After they won the Parapan American Games, they were given a place to Athens. With no world championships or other major international tournaments between then and the Paralympics, the Athens Games was the first time the world saw the USA compete. And compete, they did. They beat Slovenia convincingly 3-1 (25-20,10-25, 25-18, 25-20) to claim the bronze medal. The final two places were contested by Finland and Ukraine, where Ukraine overturned their earlier defeat by Finland in the round robin stages, to leave Finland in 6th place.

There were some attempts to put standing volleyball back into the Paralympic programme, but the event would have to re-apply through the qualification process. Sitting Volleyball was gaining a lot of momentum throughout the world. In some places, it was noted as the fastest growing inclusion sport. These trends placed the WOVD under a lot of stress in busy, but exciting times. During the following Paralympic cycle, every zone managed to run its own zonal championships.

In Europe, Bosnia and Herzegovina continue to hold onto the European crown after beating the Germans in their home country, for the 2005 European Championships, which were held in Leverkusen, Germany. Russia won the bronze medal match over Croatia, denying them of their first ever medal.

The Netherlands won the women's gold after they beat Lithuania in the final, with Slovenia finishing in third place.

2006 was the year of the triple world championships held in Roermond, Netherlands. In these championships, there were three separate volleyball tournaments; men standing volleyball, men Sitting Volleyball, and women Sitting Volleyball. In what was a well organised tournament, high spirits were around because in both men's and women's Sitting Volleyball finals, there were repeat matches to the finals two years earlier in Athens. In front of their home crowd, the Dutch women's team played faultlessly in the first two sets and showed that it was possible to take sets from the Chinese team. Then the Chinese came back and put the match went into a tie break set. After a taunting 3rd and 4th set, the home team managed to keep it together by winning the 5th set 15-12, and retained their world title.

In the men's tournament, the bronze medal match was a repeat from Athens too, whereby Egypt beat the Germans to finish 3rd place. Earlier in the day, the women's competition saw a reverse of results from the finals of the Paralympics. Supporters from Bosnia and Herzegovina came in their masses creating an immense atmosphere. The match starting time was delayed so that the crowd could settle down. There was a strong chance that Iran would do what the Netherlands did in the women's final, and the Bosnian crowd were there to make sure it wouldn't happen. Rallying their team throughout the men's final, Bosnia retained the world championships crown as they beat Iran in a spectacular match.

After the intense world championships, Iran had to immediately prepare for their zonal Parapan games, at the then called FESPIC Games, in Kuala Lumpar, Malaysia. The Sitting Volleyball competition appeared during the 1994 FEPSIC Games that were held Beijing China, and five years later in Bangkok, Thailand. Iran ran out champions on all occasions. Although the difference between the first team, Iran, and second placed China was quite large, the FESPIC Games saw the introduction of many Asian teams, in their first major international Sitting Volleyball competition.

A year later in 2007, all four zones held qualification matches for the Beijing Games. As the first three places from the world championships gave qualification to the 2008 Games, other places that had not already been allocated had to be determined by zonal competitions. This was the first time in the history of Sitting Volleyball that all zonal committees had running tournaments in the same year. The European Zone held its traditional European Championships. The African zone, in a former guise, organised its first Pan Arab Games. In the Asian Pacific zone, the women's qualification tournament took place and the American Zone had the help of the Parapan American Games to coordinate a zonal tournament.

Each zonal tournament was successful. The 2007 Asian Oceanic Championships were just for women and were held in Shanghai, China. Since China had already earned their place as host nation for the Beijing 2008 tournament, the highest placed Asian team would qualify. Additionally, the tournament attracted the USA team to take part in the Open part of the championships. The Athens Bronze medals had a disappointing World Championships in Roermond a year earlier, and were determined to get as much tournament practice as possible before they were to play in Beijing. The Shanghai Open seemed to be the perfect opportunity for this. After arranging scrimmage and friendly matches with the Chinese team, China also played USA in the final. As a result, the team that was placed 3rd overall in the tournament would qualify for the Paralympics. The two teams were Japan and Iran. Japan had previously finished ahead of the Iranian team in previous encounters, such as the 2002 and 2000 women's World Championships. However Iran had recruited the head coach of the renowned Iranian men's team to supervise the women. The battle for Beijing was set to be an exciting game, but the Japanese team prevailed, winning the match in 5 sets and a place to Beijing.

In the Americas continent, the 2007 Parapan games hosted the men's Sitting Volleyball tournament, in Rio de Janerio, Brazil. In the previous tournament, only two teams entered

Brazil and USA. In this tournament, 2 more teams entered. Canada, which was, at that time the WOVD Standing volleyball world champions and Costa Rica made up the two extra teams.

Canada has a successful record in standing volleyball and was ranked one in the world for several years. This was partly helped by a memorandum of understanding between the Canadian Amputee Sports Association and Volleyball Canada being signed in June of 1998. It was a move whereby the national federation of volleyball would include disabled volleyball into their programs, just as beach volleyball appeared. This type of move was rare, but also expected of Canadian sports bodies at that time. Since Standing volleyball was going to be taken off the programme, Dr. Robert Steadman a Canadian and President of the IPC, suggested that Standing Volleyball should look to Tennis as an organisational model. The reasons this statement was based on the way the International Tennis Federation had adopted and began administrative processes of Wheelchair Tennis.

Nevertheless, after the 2006 Triple World Championships, in Roermond, Netherlands, many of the Canadian standing players went into retirement as it appeared that their quest for Paralympic glory could only exist through the sitting game. They had either quit the sport or transferred to Sitting Volleyball, if their classification allowed them to play. The 2007 Parapan games welcomed the two new countries, and while USA had won all the group stage matches without losing a set, it wasn't until the Final that the biggest surprise of the tournament occurred. Brazil, in front of their home crowd, took the first set of the final 26-24. This was the first time USA had lost a set to another Americas team in a major international competition. They fought back to win the second and third set, but the Brazilians managed to take the game into a 5th and deciding set. With the home support, Brazil won the 5th set 15-9, and were crowed Parapan Champions earning them the right to compete in the Beijing Paralympics.

Nyiregyhaza, Hungary, was the location for the 2007 European Championships. This was the first major championships whereby a Great Britain team had played since 1992. They lost all the matches 3-0 as they learned about the international Sitting Volleyball community. The reigning World, Paralympic and European Champions continued with their unbeatable game play and put Russia in second place after 5 close sets. Russia claimed their first ever silver European medal. Germany overcame the home advantage of the Hungarian team in four sets to settle for the bronze medal. Seven teams entered the women's tournament. The Netherlands remained European Champions. Ukraine women's team, like the Russia men's team, won their first European Silver Medal, as Slovenia had to settle for the bronze. However, the main competition was about the placing of teams. As there was an absence of women teams from the African zone, then called the Afro Arab zone, and that two European teams had already qualified for Beijing from their performances at the World Championships, the highest three places in Europe would be entitled to play in Beijing. Lithuania, Latvia, and Germany were in a position to contend for two places as Ukraine reached the final, thus gaining a spot for Beijing. Lithuania also made the other semi-final match and qualified. This left Latvia and Germany competing for the final place. In a closely fought match, Latvia beat Germany 15-9 in the 5th set. After the game, there was still the theoretical possibility that Germany would qualify if, Germany beats Russia, and Russia would win their last match of the tournament against Latvia. The morning's match between Germany and Russia was a close game, but Germany did what they needed to do and that was to win. The afternoon match broke the dreams of the German players as Latvia managed to beat their neighbours in straight sets too.

The last zonal tournament of 2007 and offering the last place to the 2008 Paralympics were held in Cario, Egypt for the Pan Arab Games. The Pan Arab Games is a multi-sport event for the Arab Nations. In their 2007 sports programme, four disability sports were included in the multi-sport tournament. Since Egypt had already qualified for Beijing, following their 3rd place in the world championships, the team that finished second would have been awarded a place in the 2008 Paralympics. Iraq fulfilled this criterion as Libya and Jordan competed for the first time, and Morocco finished in third place.

2008-2012

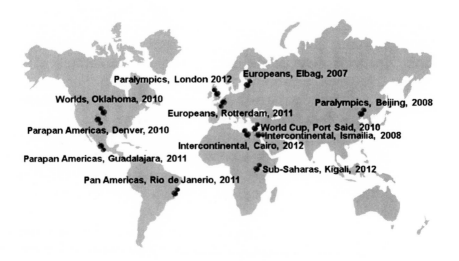

8. Map of competition venues 2008-2012

3.2.6 **2008 – 2012 Two tiered Sitting Volleyball**

The WOVD organised the first Intercontinental Cup just before the Beijing Games, in Ismalia, Egypt. For teams, officials and administrations, it was the opportunity to make final preparations for the Summer Games. This was the first time the Iranian men team were able to play against other teams in major international competitions. The eventual winners were Iran, with Russia second, and Bosnia and Herzegovina, third. In the women's tournament, the Netherlands beat Slovenia in the Final, and the USA team finished third.

Later that year, the 2008 Paralympics took place in Beijing, China. A new ball was introduced to all volleyball competitions. It was designed to make the rallies last longer because the ball could not be hit so hard, and yet it would be easier to control in the defence. Also the amount of air floating from the service was designed to have been reduced, and making it easier to receive. In the men's tournament, Iran was looking to overturn the recent run of the Bosnians. The two teams faced each other in the final, and Iran swept Bosnia 3-0. Russia won the bronze medal after beating Egypt in the fifth set. In the women's competition, the host nation dominated throughout the entire tournament. In December 2007, there was the tragic and unexpected death of the Chinese Head coach, and their competition schedule was put aside as the team regrouped. Any doubts about the new coaching staff were reassured as they won every match without dropping a set. The semi-final match between USA and The Netherlands was a closely fought game. USA were pushed to a fifth set but managed to win 15-10. After their shock semi-final defeat, the Dutch women bounced back to claim the bronze medal.

Eleven men's and eight women's teams travelled to Elbag, Poland for the 2009 European Championships. This was the first time a Great Britain team had won a major international tournament match for over twenty years. They beat Greece once in the pool games and another time in the classification matches to finish in 10th place. Other teams competed for the right to compete at the 2010 World Championships. Bosnia and Herzegovina, Russia, and Germany took the medals respectively, and in the top three from the women's tournament, were the same placing as the 2007 European Championships; Netherland – 1st; Ukraine – 2nd; Slovenia – 3rd.

Pan American qualification for the world championships began in Denver, USA in the early part of 2010. Since Sitting Volleyball falls under the remit of the USA Volleyball Association and not a separate, disability sports organisation, the role of Sitting Volleyball in social inclusion plays a strong role. This tournament was held in conjunction with the Colorado Crossroads tournament, whereby 15 categories of around 1000 teams between 12-18 year old youth played over two weekends. The profile of Sitting Volleyball to the volleyball community in the USA, was increased as young teams, coaches, managers and media were able to support their home team, USA and for some, be exposed to Sitting Volleyball for the first time. The purpose of the tournament was to give the right for top two teams to compete in the 2010 World Championships. USA, Brazil and Canada fielded a team for both men and women competitions. The final placing from the men's tournament was the same for the women's. The US team overcame their recent loss to Brazil in the 2007 Parapan American Games in the final by winning 3-0. The first appearance of a women's team from Canada was a courageous one, although they did not manage to win a set throughout the entire tournament, they gained much experience with major competitions.

Less than two weeks after the Pan American Championships, the USA teams travelled to Port Said, Egypt, to compete in the World Cup. This was the new name for the Intercontinental cup, which was held in Ismailia, Egypt in 2008, and acted as a warm up tournament for the world championships. Due to the close proximity of the tournament, Algeria featured a team for the first time in major tournaments and finished in 8th place ahead of Great Britain who finished in last place. The absence of Bosnia and Herzegovina from the tournament prevented a pre-Worlds showdown between the top two teams in the world and the much anticipated match would only take place at the World Championships. Not surprisingly, Iran won the World Cup, with Germany taking silver. Kazakhstan's best ever finish was at the world cup, but they just lost out to the hosts, Egypt, in the 3rd/4th play-off. In the women's tournament, the USA team continued to improve their results by beating the Netherlands in the final in four sets, and Slovenia finished ahead of Russia, also in four sets, to claim third place. Egypt brought together, for the first time, a women's team, but were unable to make any progress as they lost every match and often finding it hard to attack and averaged 25 points in each match.

The third major tournament in 2010 was the World Championships. Originally, there were intentions for another triple world championship, following the success in Roermond, Netherlands. However, the focus for the world championships would be just on Sitting Volleyball as standing volleyball would have its own tournament. This meant there was the possibility for more teams to enter, than it was originally anticipated. To date, this was largest ever international Sitting Volleyball tournament. A total of 35 teams, 21 men and 12 women, arrived in Denver for a week long tournament. The men's competition was first divided into 4 preliminary pools, and the top three teams from each pool went into Division-A for the final stages, and the lower teams would then be placed into a Division-B tournament. The same structure was also organised for the women's competition, however there were only two pools of 6 teams, and the top 4 teams of each pool made up an eight team Division-A. In the men's A-Division, Iran met with Bosnia and Herzegovina in a close final and won the game eventually in 5 sets. Iran took the first two sets but lost the third and fourth sets. In the fifth set Iran held on to reclaim their world championships gold. Egypt managed to retain their 3rd place from the 2006 World Championships after beating Paralympic Bronze medallists, Russia, in the 3rd/4th play-off game. In the B-Division, Kazakhstan beat Morocco to claim the B-Division gold medal match, and Hungary took the bronze.

In the women's tournament, despite having home advantage over the Paralympic Champions, China swept the young USA team in 3 sets to take their first world championships title. The World Championships in Oklahoma, USA were the first major tournament that the Dutch women's team did not take home a medal, as they lost to Ukraine in the fight for 3rd place. In Division-B, Brazil beat Japan to claim top place, and Great Britain received its first ever women's Sitting Volleyball medal by beating Canada for the bronze medal. This game was also the first major international match that a Great Britain women's team had ever won, while the Canadians will have to wait a bit longer for glory.

Formerly known as FESPIC Games, the final major international tournament in 2010 was the Asian Para Games, held in Guangzhou, China. Other than the 2008 Games, this was the first time a men's and women's tournament co-existed in Asia. In the men's tournament, there were 8 teams. The newest teams were Thailand and Myanmar, who finished in 8th and 7th place respectively. Iran continued with its dominance, China took the second place, while Iraq finished in 3rd place. The women's tournament saw a debut entry by Pakistan. Since China had already qualified from the World Championships, the focus on who would qualify for London was on the semi-final between Iran and Japan. As expected, it was a close encounter. Japan came back from behind to win the match and thus securing qualification for the London Games.

2011 was the year of qualification for the European and American zones. Places for the 2012 games were becoming very competitive in the men's European Zone. Bosnia and Herzegovina had qualified from the world championships, and the best finishing European team other than the Bosnians would qualify. As the tournament turned out, Germany came out top in their group, but eventually lost to Russia in the semi-final in straight sets. With Bosnia taking the other final place, Russia, had qualified for the Paralympics, and were contending for the title of European Champion. Russia started off strongly by taking the first set. Bosnia and Herzegovina regrouped to take the next three sets and continued to dominate European men's Sitting Volleyball. In the women's tournament, Ukraine had already won its ticket to the London Games after they won the bronze in the 2010 World Championships. They faced the Netherlands in the final as both teams entered the match unbeaten throughout the tournament. After the Netherlands had lost its title as World Championships winners, they also lost the title of European Champions when they collapsed against Ukraine in the 3rd and 4th set to lose 3-1, but had got a place for London. Russia won its first ever women's medal after beating Slovenia 3-1 to claim the bronze medal.

For some unknown reasons, the Parapan American Games in Guadalajara, Mexico hosted only the men's Sitting Volleyball competition. Since there needed to be a qualification process, the American's zone set up a Pan American Qualifiers tournament just for women in Rio de Janeiro, Brazil. In the four team tournament, Columbia entered for their first time, while the rest of the tournament there weren't many surprises. USA had already qualified for London after they won the silver from the world championships. This left the zonal place for the Paralympics to come from either Brazil or Canada. Brazil had won the gold B-Division tournament in the world championships, and they demonstrated their superiority against the Canadians by qualifying for the final against the US team, and a place for London. The men's tournament was held in conjunction with the Parapan American Games. To demonstrate the development of the sport throughout the continent, the number of teams increased as Columbia and Mexico played its first tournament, both finishing ahead of Costa Rica. In a similar way, Brazil, USA, and Canada took the 1st, 2nd, and 3rd places respectively.

An additional slot for the men's competition in the Paralympics was made for teams that could qualify from the Sub-Sahara Region. This would mean that Sitting Volleyball has 10 men's team and only 8 women's teams. As the Paralympic Games have a limited number of places that can be allocated to sports, when the agreement came for more male teams, it came at a price of reducing the number of players in a team from 12 players to 11 players. This is a modification to the rules of the game, and although it is great to see the development in Sub-Sahara, other teams would have to sacrifice a 12 man strong team by axing one player to allow for two more teams.

The Sub-Sahara competition was the first competition in 2012 for the remaining places for the London Games. Held in Rwanda, the inaugural Sub-Sahara qualification tournament took place during the end of February. In the years leading up to these championships, many Sub-Saharan countries had been getting experience from WOVD instructors, international coaches and sport development officers. A high quality event took place with the sponsorship from UKSport, an organisation that helped pay for some legacy work from the 2012 games. The hosts Rwanda came out winners, beating Kenya in the Final, and Uganda finished 3rd after beating Burundi in the play-off game, with DCR Congo in last place.

A few weeks later, and due to politics around North Africa, there were many weeks of uncertainty as to whether an Intercontinental Cup could be played in Cairo. In this tournament, the best placed team from the North African region would qualify for the London Games. Fortunately, the tournament was unaffected from the recent political rife. The three teams and their zonal places were 1st. Egypt, 2nd. Morocco, and 3rd. Libya. The Intercontinental cup served as the final major championships prior to the London games. 12 men's teams played from around the world, and 6 women. In the men's tournament, Iran came out first after beating hosts Egypt in the finals, and Russia took the bronze. In the women's tournament, the USA team did not enter, as China won the gold convincingly as they beat Ukraine in the final, and this tournament was the second bronze medal for the Russian team as they beat Slovenia in the 3rd/4th play-off game.

The London 2012 Games were a major step forward in the advancement of the Paralympics. It was the first time that city bids for being awarded the games required a campaign that included both Olympic and Paralympic plans. The London games also allowed a 'day pass' ticketing scheme where the ticket holders could see a multitude of Paralympic events. During the early rounds and qualification matches, Sitting Volleyball was visible for day passes, however the finals for both men and women were ticket only matches. This was the first time Great Britain competed in the Paralympics for both men and women, although the majority of media focus was on the Rwandan team. The seeding system placed Great Britain, the host nation, as first seed, which meant that world number one and two would play against each other in the pool play. There were also ten teams in the men's competition and eight women's teams. When it was agreed to have two extra men's teams, one from the Sub-Sahara region and another could compete in London, the athlete quota had already been reached, and this was the first and last time teams were told that would be a maximum of 11 players per squad, even though the rules specify a maximum of 12 players.

The women's competition was mixture of youth and experience with the oldest player at 55 years old and the youngest 14 years old. The group stages went according to the rankings of the world championships two years earlier with the top four teams qualifying for the semi-finals. However, Brazil made progress by taking sets against China and USA and was set to challenge for the 5th place against Slovenia, which they did in four sets. China managed to hold out the American team for a second Paralympic final to take their third consecutive gold in Sitting Volleyball. Great Britain's debut ended without winning a set throughout the tournament as they lost out to Japan in the final 7-8th placement match.

The men's competition had 10 teams which meant that it was possible for teams to play a round of quarter-finals before final placement matches. Since each pool comprised of 10 teams, the top four would play in quarter finals, and the bottom two would play for the 9th-10th places. In an all-African match, Rwanda claimed the title of second best team in Africa as they came back from 1 set and 25-24 behind to win their first set in the competition and then on to win the match. In the other games, Iran won their group by beating Bosnia, and other teams were very competitive with 3-2 results in the final placement games, including Germany taking bronze over Russia. The men's final was eventually won by Bosnia, who managed to win their second goal in three Paralympics after being 1 set and 18-16 behind. Great Britain's only win was against Morocco in the group stages and finished in 8th place behind China. Brazil had to overcome Egypt for 5th place.

3.3 **Alternatives**

Since 2008, there has been an immense increase in interest in playing Sitting Volleyball at major competitions. This is an increasing trend in the number of countries playing the sport. It has certainly established itself as the number one alternative form of volleyball for the disabled. Despite the ease to playability of the German version of sitzball, the game is too dissimilar to volleyball that it has been difficult to become the popular game for amputees.

In brief, sitzball is a combination between tennis and volleyball. The net is set at 1m high and is a band across a 8m wide court that separates the 10m court length. Between each shot, the ball is allowed to bounce once. A maximum of three touches are allowed. Lifting the body to play the ball is permitted. There are only 5 players per team. The rally commences from team passing the ball for an attack. Games are played by scoring the most amounts of points in a given time limit. Since these rules are vastly different from volleyball, it has some very complex set of tactics. Furthermore, the game is governed by time, and bouncing of the ball is allowed between team members when composing an attack, so scoring against opponents can often be dictated by the way the other teams play the ball on their side of the court.

Standing volleyball is an official sport of the WOVD, and has regular world cup championships. Although it is no longer in the Paralympic sports programmes, the 2011 world cup in Cambodia had sell-out crowds in the final between Germany and Cambodia. A sport that is very popular in Cambodia, the majority of players enjoy the standing game so much, that do not play the game sitting on the floor. Whereas, after winning the 2006 Triple World Championships Standing volleyball Tournament, in Roermond, Netherlands, Canada dissolved the national team and focused on the sitting game. The standing game has more levels of classification. It is like other disability team sports, whereby teams cannot have more than a number of classified points playing on the court at any one time.

Two new versions of volleyball for the disabled are currently under review. Beach standing volleyball is played by three players and has been popularised in Germany. The WOVD have organised a number of tournaments, and it is likely to gain more popularity as a sport for the disabled. This has the potential to reach the Paralympics in the future. The other version of beach volleyball is beach Sitting Volleyball. Although this game has been tried in and around Europe, players have found several problems with the game. It is difficult to move in the sand without getting sand into the eyes. The court is often either too small or too big to make spectacular rallies. If Sitting Volleyball is designed to be fair, by ensuring players have their lower body or back in contact with the floor when playing the ball, checking for this on sand is difficult. Much sand moves around, and players may find themselves moving to positions of sand that are higher, or position the opponents on lower parts of sand. These disadvantages could then make players lift from the ground more, however, knowing where the ground is already difficult when using sand. The alternative to beach Sitting Volleyball is to play on a hard court, nearby the beach. Using the beach volleyball, players play on harder surfaces where they can benefit from exercise in the sun, and also eliminate the risks of sand pollution and regulations formed by the game's lifting policy.

4 RULES OF THE GAME

The rules of the game determine how the game can be played, and are abided by. The referee corps has the responsibility to reinforce good sportsmanship and maintain fairness amongst the teams. Referees in Sitting Volleyball are usually trained to first understand the art of refereeing volleyball games before they subsequently learn the different ways they need to adopt for the sitting game. The refereeing corps consists of referees, line judges and scorers. There are two main refereeing responsibilities. The first referee makes the overall decision and can overrule any other decisions made from the other officials. Teams can protest against decisions, but only after the game has ended. The second referee's main role is to support the first referee. Although their responsibilities are less than the first referee, if they deem the first referee is not in the right position to see an infringement of the rules, they can have the authority to interfere with play and make calls that affect the way points are scored. The first and second referee are often opposite each other, whereby the first referee is standing by the post and is quite static, while the second referee moves around the opposite post depending on what they are doing in relation to the game play, the position of the first referee, the ball placement and ability to control the rest of the court.

Line judges have limited responsibilities. They have lines to monitor and assist the referees in making their decision by indicating whether the ball has landed in or out of court. They will also have to watch the attack shot, as it might have touched the block on the way out the court, for which they use a special signal to the referees. They are also in a position whereby they can see if the ball has landed on the court, when the referees cannot see clearly if the ball has touched the floor. Sometimes the referee's view of angle and the position of the players in relation to the ball may obscure the floor contact. Since line judges are positioned by the lines, they are also in the best position to determine whether players are outside or inside the court when play commences. They can also help the first referee to determine if the ball crosses over the net, inside or outside the crossing space. The crossing space is an extended vertical line that extends above and below the antenna. The antenna is a pole that points perpendicular to the floor directly above the outer part of the side line. There is a rule that states, "The ball must cross the opponent's court through the crossing space". There is also the issue of recovery of the ball that goes outside the crossing space and into the other side of the hall. However, it is an extremely rare situation for Sitting Volleyball, partly due to the mobility issues of the athletes.

The scorers have the responsibility to record the score of the teams, and adjudicate the correct serving order, proper libero exchanges, the number of substitutions and controlling time outs. Under the quick substitution rule, the scoring table members will notify the referees that a substitution will take place, once the player enters the substitution zone. The substitution zone is defined by the line extensions beyond the attack line. That is the lines two metres from the centre line and the net. Once a substitute enters this part of the field, they are indicating that they would like to substitute a player. At this time, the scorer makes an audible sound that will notify the referees of a legal interruption of the game, and that at least one of six substitutions per team is being taken in the set.

The scorers, line judges, and the referees form the referee corps. In major competitions, there are 4 line judges, with the main responsibility on the line in front of them. They are numbered one through to four, beginning with the line judge to the right of the first referee, going anti clockwise. In other words, the line judge, with the main responsibility of the baseline to the left of the referee, is line judge 4, while the line judge whose main responsibility is to monitor the sideline in front of the first referee is line judge 1. Illustrations of positions of the officials can be found in Volleyball rule books.

In organised tournaments with sufficient amount of officials, there are at least two scorers controlling the score sheet. The first scorer completes the main score sheet, that gets submitted to the competition organiser, and the second scorer acts as the assistant to the first scorer, and controls the score board, substitution alerts and technical time outs. Other scorers maybe in charge of maintaining electronic scoreboards, but they are only observing the assistant scorer's score. A libero scorer is often needed too, as this helps with the exchange of liberos in the back court. Another official may also be nominated to the scorer's table to monitor classification of the teams. Their responsibility is to make sure that teams are not putting players onto the court that make the team ineligible due to classification restrictions.

Under the current Sitting Volleyball rules, teams are allowed to have two players with a minimal disability classification in the squad, however, only one minimal disability player is allowed to play on court any one time. Similar to the libero rule, whereby teams can have two liberos in the team, and only one libero can enter the court. The restriction on the types of players on the court is to promote fairness amongst teams as well as adherence to the rules of the game.

For future considerations of the classification of Sitting Volleyball team compositions, classification may be altered. There have been discussions whereby players are either just disabled or not disabled. Some classification experts have compared minimally disabled players with disabled players and have found that the minimal disability players tend to be the strongest players in the squad, which would mean, having more than one minimal disabled player on the court, would give that team a lot of strength. However, other experts have contested those findings and oppose those suggestions, requesting that further research in their area is needed before making drastic changes to the classification rules. Whether the classification rule is changed or not, the issue of classification will always be a contentious issue surrounding disability sports and over time, there may be differences to suit the adaptable changes to the types of disabilities entering the sport at development, elite and junior levels.

4.1 Differences between standing and Sitting Volleyball

Rules of Sitting Volleyball are based on slight modifications to the indoor game rules. To avoid confusion, in this text, indoor volleyball is referred to as the game played by non-disabled. Standing volleyball refers to the indoor game played by disabled athletes and governed by the WOVD. There is a usual tendency to adopt the same rule changes from the indoor game to the sitting game. Exceptions are made when the changes from the standing game cannot be applied to the sitting game. Strictly speaking, there are 16 rule differences between the sitting and the indoor game. Much of the rules are similar, and can be broken down into five main differences, these being; 1. Height of the net; 2. Court dimensions; 3. Service block/attack; 4. Buttocks determining plays; and 5. The joust and penetration.

4.1.1 Height of the net

The standing volleyball court rules place the height of the net at 2.43m for men and 2.24m for women. The average attack height of world class men volleyball players is; 3.43m and for women it is 3.01m. The difference between the average spike heights for men over the height of the net for men is therefore 99.91cm. The women, who have less power output, are actually only jumping, on average 76.83cm over the height of the net. In Sitting Volleyball, players have to remain in contact with the floor, and therefore the height of the net is set lower, whereby the net height for the men is 1.15m, and for women it is 1.05m.

To put things into perspective, to be able to play Sitting Volleyball like the standing players, men players need to be reaching the ball at 2.15m and for women, their contact point of a spike should be around 1.80m. Therefore the sitting players will have to have very long limbs and tall body torsos in order to reach such heights. Latest anthropological measurements of players indicate the average contact point height for men is 1.49m and 1.39m for women. The difference between the two genders is the same as the height of the net changes between men and women.

This height has remained the same since the first set of codified rules for Sitting Volleyball was written. Whereas the average height difference between men and women around the world is 12.22cm, by rounding the height difference to 15cm might have been too excessive, as the tallest female nation (The Netherlands) is the only nation whereby the average difference in height between men and women is over 15cm. The net height difference of just 10cm can make the women's game more attractive than the game played by men. The extra 2cm of average height gained by women over the difference in net height could also be compensated for the lower velocity speeds through striking the ball by women. This level of compensation places more emphasis on the placement of the ball and control of the court than of power, hard hitting and reducing reaction times of the defending player. Furthermore, the actual height difference between people playing Sitting Volleyball has been reported to be 10cm, which validates the difference between the genders, irrespective of the world-wide national average height differences among genders.

4.1.2 **Court Dimensions**

Sitting Volleyball court sizes are rectangular, with each side being 6m wide by 5m long, so that the entire volleyball court is 10m by 6m. This is 37% less court space than the standing volleyball court, which is 18m by 9m. The longest distance from the top of the net to the corner of the court is 61% less in Sitting Volleyball than in the standing game. The difference is the same in both the men and women height net.

These distances were calculated based on playing the ball from one corner of the diagonal to the other, hence making the furthest distance, and then combined with the height at the top of the net. While the men's net height standing volleyball court makes the longest distance possible at 13.18m, the women distance at 13.08m, the sitting game distances are 7.89m and 7.88m for men and women, respectively. The ratios between the genders are both 61%. Although these distances cannot be played by the actual player, because either the antenna interference, ball clipping the top of the net cord, or the amount of spin generated by the attacker, the distances and difference put into perspective a standardised comparison between the two types of courts.

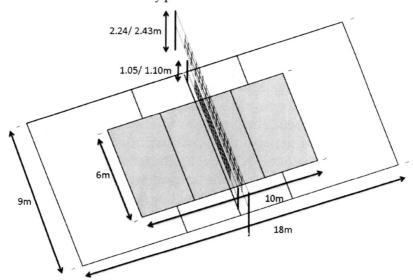

9. Sitting Volleyball Court in relation to an indoor court.

The attack line is placed at 2m from the centre line. Its main purpose is to prevent all round dominance by a singular player on the team, and enhances team cohesion. Teams will find that attacking from the back of the court to be less advantageous than attacking in the front zone, so when the player rotates to the backrow for half of the game, another player has the possibility to attack in the front zone. While the ratio between the standing court of 3m for the attack line remains the same at 61% between the indoor and Sitting Volleyball court, there is a 0.001m difference that sitting players have less ratio to attack for a backrow attack than standing players. These minor differences are so slight, they are not significant enough to have the dimensions of the court recalibrated to the nearest millimetre, rather than by metres.

In the early part of the 21st century, there were some tests conducted among teams to see if the court could be extended to 6m long. The court would then resemble a standing court, as each side would have a square. The primary focus was based to see if attacking players would make fewer errors in hitting the ball out of the court. A result from several years of elite sports analysis that saw a high percentage of attacks being hit out of the court. After some testing competitions, and feedback sessions, the teams and evaluators concluded that the existing court dimensions were suitable for the game play. It is the responsibility of the attacking team to find ways of scoring by attacking inside the court, rather than out of the court. Therefore, the court dimensions remain the same at 10m x 6m since the game was first codified in the 1960s.

Teams that practice and want to utilise the existing indoor volleyball court lines can find two main ways of setting up a Sitting Volleyball court. With the dimensions of the sitting court being 6m wide, it is the same length as the backrow zone of an indoor court. The sitting court almost fits perfectly into a volleyball court, if the service line wasn't 50cm further away from the indoor volleyball side-lines. Matches played on this half court system might have to mark the line extensions in another colour to that which is used for the indoor volleyball court lines. Different colour lines can help avoid confusion of which of the two lines is actually the back line. Otherwise, the half court system only requires minimal modification to the existing volleyball court lines. Therefore, two simultaneous games can take place on one volleyball court as the other backrow zone is used for another Sitting Volleyball game. However, in order to use the court in this way, two volleyball net and post systems need to be fitted so games can be played that way.

If a court does not have post and net fittings along the side of the court, it is safer to use the existing indoor volleyball fittings and move the court closer to one of the side-lines. In this way, three of the Sitting Volleyball lines need to be marked, and net tension at one end is required as the existing system can hold a net with sufficient tension on the other end. Games that use the side-line can have the referee's position close enough to the where the action is and still position be in the middle of the court.

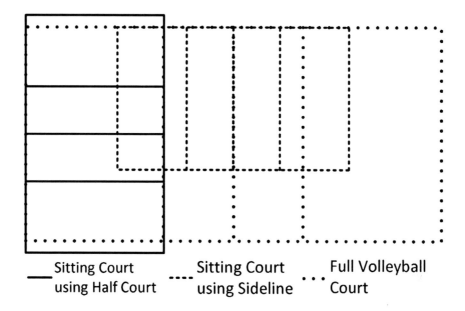

___ Sitting Court using Half Court

_ _ _ Sitting Court using Sideline

• • • Full Volleyball Court

10. Converting Indoor Court for Sitting Volleyball

4.1.3 Service block/attack

Depending on the team's preferences, they may choose to have service blockers. The service blocker is designated to block off the low, fast and powerful serve that are directed to a certain part of the court. To make this rule simple and without getting into the complexity of defining what constitutes a block or not, an additional rule enables a front court attack of the serve. Therefore, an attacking motion of the ball as well as blocking the ball from service is permitted. In the standing game, both these rules were taken out during the 1960s.

The blockers in the sitting game are positioned closer to the server so that a significant portion of the court that a blocker can reduce, should the ball be hit hard, fast and low over the net. In order to prevent servers from scoring service aces, teams may position their players that would best help their reception unit as well as form some sort of attack against the serve.

The rule about attacking a serve also takes away the advantage of slow balls being sent over the top of the block, and landing directly behind the blocker. Since blockers can then become attackers, and since movement is often restricted by the receivers, the permission to attack the serve often makes the server serve aggressively against the reception unit, avoiding the block and potential drop shots that go over and behind the block.

4.1.4 Buttocks determining plays

Sitting on the floor has many benefits and many disadvantages. In most cases it can mean that there are vast arrays of players that can play the game. People without and with lower limbs can play Sitting Volleyball without the extra expense of wheelchairs and the risk of injury. However, in the standing game, players can jump and move about using their legs, and in the rules of the sitting game, the buttocks replace the legs.

The buttocks are largely defined as an area of the human that stretches from the top of the back to the very extremity of their back, including their backside, or in Latin, the 'glutimus maximus'.

In order to create fairness among the players, one major difference between standing and Sitting Volleyball is playing the ball while in contact with the floor. While standing volleyball encourages high vertical reaches, mainly consisting of jumping, the sitting player must be constantly touching the floor. Since different types of disabilities can play together, the fairest way would be to limit the buttocks as the point of contact with the floor when playing the ball. An infringement of this is known as 'lifting'.

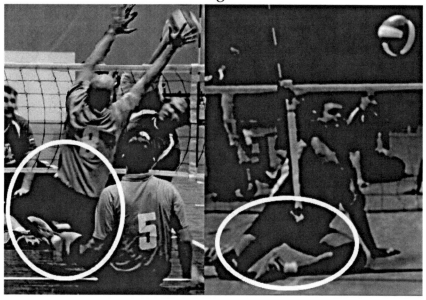

11. Lifting while Blocking (left) and Attacking (right)

Lifting occurs when more than one part of the buttocks is not in contact with the floor when playing the ball. This is a hard thing for the referee to decide upon. Technically speaking, players are not allowed to play the ball while lifting their body off from the floor. This would generate advantages over the opponents when reaching for the ball, instead of keeping contact with the ground. There are five shots, whereby the player can be called for lifting. During service, receiving, setting, attacking and blocking.

During service, the player may be lifting when serving. They will tend to do this, when trying to generate a powerful serve. In order to generate a lot of power on the serve, the server may want to use forward momentum when serving. In order to do this, as the player is moving forwards, they may find that they are actually moving off the ground when striking the ball. Players also want to hit the ball from as high up as possible and this too can cause the server to lift themselves momentarily when serving.

The act of receiving the ball from an underarm pass in front of the player can often be interpreted as lifting the body, instead of moving forwards to play the ball. In the modern game, this is becoming quite rare to see, as a lot of players start to position them closer to the net and play the reception shot with an overarm shot. However, some teams may still be positioned quite far back of the court and end up lunging forwards for the short service. The lunging motion could prompt lifting of their buttocks.

Many setters will try to push themselves forwards and upwards to move the ball to the desired position on the court for the attack. In teams where there are specialist setters, they may find themselves moving to get to the ball whilst under a lot of pressure before they have to the push the ball towards the designated place for the attacker. Setters have other possible infringements that can happen at the time of contacting the ball. Their contact is very important and often they will contact the ball at least once in the possible three contacts. When formulating an attack, the setter may be called up from the referee on several handling faults as well as lifting.

The attacker can lift when trying to contact the ball at a higher position, or trying to generate more force when striking the ball. As with the service lifting fault, the attacker wants to strike the ball with as much power and accuracy as possible. In order to generate power, the attacker may find their forward momentum lifting them up when contacting the ball. Furthermore, the attacker has a better angle of attack when playing the ball from a higher contact point, as such, if the ball is beyond their reach, the player may find themselves lifting.

Blocking can be a bit more technical. Generally speaking, in a one-on-one situation, the blocker is trying to prevent the attacking shot from entering their own court. The block forms the first line of defence and it can be considered as an attacking shot. As an aggressive shot, contacting the ball higher can be more beneficial over the attacker, and blockers may find themselves lifting while in the blocking action (see figure 11). Sometimes, there is the collective block. During a collective block, irrespective of whether the player who touches the ball had or had not lifted, should another member of that collective block lift, then the team is penalised.

Finally, the buttocks not only play an important role during the time playing the ball, the rules also use the buttocks as the determinant of player positions on the court. There are six positions on a volleyball court, starting in position 1 in the back right corner away from the net. Rotating anti-clockwise to subsequent positions 2, which is front right, position 3, front middle and position 4 in the front left. Position 5 is back left and position 6 is back middle.

In the standing game, a player commits a foot fault when they have either stepped on the line during the execution of serve, or if they are not serving, are outside the court when a rally starts. The same rule has been modified in Sitting Volleyball, but is determined by the player's buttocks. The positions of players are determined by the feet being closer to the centre line or side line in the standing game. In other words, the player in position one must have their outside foot more closer to the right side line than the player in position six and must have their back foot more closer to the end line than the player in position two. In Sitting Volleyball these rules are still enforced, but instead of using the feet as determinants of positions, the buttocks are used. Player's hands, arms and legs can be in any position in or out of the court without being penalised. The referee is only concerned with the position of the buttocks in relation to other players and the court.

4.1.5 **The Joust and penetration.**

A lot of the Sitting Volleyball rules follow rule changes that occur in the standing game. There are some cases where this cannot happen. An example of this is the change in the joust rule in 2009. A joust occurs above the net between two or more opposing players that forces the ball to become stationary. The new rules in indoor volleyball suggest that jousts are no longer called from simultaneous contacts between two opponents. The outcome of the joust would continue until the rally ended. In Sitting Volleyball, a joust may last too long, since both players are sitting on the floor. Once players are sitting comfortably at the net, and the ball comes towards the net, both opponents may end up reaching for the ball. This simultaneous contact will end up as a joust. In standing volleyball, the only way to reach above the net is through jumping. The consequence of jumping is landing, and hands would end up lower than the net, and thus end the joust. In other words, the joust in the standing game can only last for a short moment. Whereas, in the sitting game, since players are not allowed to lift their buttocks from the floor when playing the ball, and since they can reach beyond the top of the net, there are many possibilities that the ball becomes stationary and therefore a joust stops the movement of the ball. At this point, the referees would look to end the joust and replay the point.

Similarly, the interference under the net is often seen in the sitting game. In the standing game, it can be obvious to see the entire foot under the net. The infringement is made based on penetration into the opponent's court. Some sitting players have legs, and the only way their bodies will allow them to be close to the net for blocking or attacking is to put parts of the legs under the net, and into the opponent's court. In this way, the sitting game has modified the rule from disallowing the entire foot from penetrating under the net, to the entire hand over the centre line as penetration. It is very rare that players have their entire hand under the net and get penalised for it. It is more likely that players are caught interfering with the opponent's play above the net.

4.2 **Protests**

The rules of the game are an important part of the game that all people, players, coaches, managers, referees, and spectators should be able to understand. In fact, the first rule, relating to sportsmanship, states that players must know and abide by the official Sitting Volleyball rules.

Often, misinterpretation of the rules can cause confusion between teams and the refereeing corps. Sometimes, incorrect decisions are made and until there are sufficient testing from recall technology, like the hawk-eye for line calls, slow motion detection cameras for touches off the block, motion sensors for net interference rules, the sole judgement and interpretations by the refereeing corps has to be accepted as the final decision and the point should stand.

Teams that find they were left without justice from one or two calls by the officials can often be found to blame themselves. Teams have to achieve 25 points before their opponents, with a two point cushion. There are plenty of opportunities for teams to get ahead of their opponents, and small mistakes by the referees, need not be a problem. Although, in the heat of the moment, players are often caught up with the belief that they have won the point and try to convince officials of their conviction.

Spectators may also be left confused with what they see and what the referee ends up calling. The most common interruption of play in Sitting Volleyball is the 'lifting' call. Often spectators cannot see the players' buttocks from lifting from the floor. If there is an exciting rally, and if the ball is still in play, it does not make much sense to the spectator that one of the players has lifted. If a ball lands in the court, or if the ball goes out, and the spectators cannot see the infringing player from lifting, then, when calls that go the opposite way, the audience are often left bemused by the decisions of the referees.

Similar effects can be noticed by the referee, who sees the ball touching the fingertips of the blocker, and the ball landing far out from the court. Although the ball has landed very far from the court, the ball should be considered as landed out of bounds and the point goes to the defending team. However, the referee may consider it a fault of the defending team, because the referee had seen the ball touching the block as it flew out of court. Sometimes, referees will overrule the line-judge, but in most cases, in disputable situations, the referee will ask the concerning line-judge to approach the first referee and to speak with that referee about the decision. Without the possibility of action replay, all those involved in the outcome of the point; the players, opponents, line judges, and referees, will have to recall what were the course of actions with precision before the referees make their decision.

The use of action replay technology is still under development in the indoor volleyball game. With the introduction to hi-tech equipment, some competitions have tried a 'challenge' approach used by teams, with the aim to reverse the decisions made by referees. Slow motion action replay and an extra official then become integral parts of the game, but the process causes interruptions to game flow, although correct decisions are made. In some cases, this has proven to be an effective means of ensuring the right decision has been made so that the correct team that wins the rally is awarded a point. However, this is only limited to the technology available and the users of the equipment. When there becomes too much reliance on technology, the camera must be placed in a position related to the ball, line, net, antenna and the fingers of the blocker. Slow motion cameras with sufficient high definition are required to demonstrate clearly whether the ball has landed in or out of the court, if the net was infringed by the player, or if the net touched the player. A balance between the amount of time taken to interrupt play and adjudicating the correct decision has to be made, whereby the overall flow of the game continues. In some cases, teams may make challenge requests for very clear decisions and use that time for a time out, whereby players sort out their strategies for the next point, irrespective of the outcome of the challenge.

For Sitting Volleyball, the camera used for observing lifting, will first require referees to be able to call inappropriate lifting calls, thus risking the flow of the game, with regular interruptions, and then the use of the camera whereby it is possible to observe the lower body and the contact point of the ball. Teams cannot request the referee to check an infringement that the referees have not called. This might cause a lot of confusion between points, and too much time taken to discuss between players and referees, at which point in the rally, did they miss the infringement. As this can become confusing and wasting time, such rules would seem virtually impossible to recall based on video evidence.

The lifting rule can occur many times during a rally, and more often than not, players will notice themselves whether they are lifting or if the decision was incorrect. Players will also notice if they have touched the ball during the block action. In most cases, the players will generate a small protest towards the referee's decisions, irrespective of whether they have or have not made such errors. Players may find that they are under immense stress by their coaches and teams, which could induce the feeling that they would naturally feel that they had not caused such faults. The pressure placed on players could mean that they are substituted by another player, and it is very rare to find a player who does not want to play.

Some other teams will make a collective protest to the referee's decisions, such as indicating to the referee that the opponent has touched the ball, when their player strikes the ball out of the court. They might also collectively cheer, even though they might have seen or felt something occurring on the court that was a fault and they should have lost the point. Under most circumstances, the team morale is important, and at the end of every point, teams will often gather together and try to convince the referees, opponents, the spectators, even themselves that they have won the point.

Officially, protests should only go through the captain on the court. While each team has their own game captain, that is the person who goes for the toss, the court captain is the player who is the captain of the team on the court if the game captain is not currently playing. The rules state that only the game captain can communicate with the first referee. This also includes the interaction between the coach and the first referee. Strictly speaking, the first referee will have to speak to the captain to communicate with the coach. In sportsmanship conduct cases, often the referee will speak to the captain and ask them to relay the message to the coach. Failing this communication, the referee can communicate with the coach with warnings and penalty cards. The process of penalising all other players is also the same as communicating via the captain. In a situation where a player, who is not the captain, is called up by the referee for lifting, the player may at first want to protest to say that they did not lift. It is normal for humans to defend themselves when they are accused of something that they have not done. However, if that player were to persist in protesting the referee's decision without going through the game captain, and behaving in an unsportsmanlike manner, that player may then be sanctioned with a warning or penalty. Even though they did not infringe on the first ruling, unsportsmanlike conduct is not tolerated. However, due to their subsequent actions and reactions to the referee, they were penalised due to unsportsmanlike conduct.

Although this process many seem a little tiresome at times, it is an effective means of controlling the court, players and coaches. Referees do not purposely intend on giving out penalties to team members, but sometimes they need to sanction players for misbehaviour or continued troublesome actions.

4.3 **Summary of the rules**

Without the fairness governed with what is written in the rules and the enforcement of these by the referees, teams may end up with an unfair advantage in a game that was adapted to play with equality among the players. Sitting Volleyball modified its rule from volleyball so that many types of abilities could play together and have an equal chance of winning a game.

Since Sitting Volleyball is an adaptation of the indoor volleyball, it follows the rule changes in the standing game, and modifies it to the sitting game. There are 16 rule differences written between the two rules books, although the differences can appear in 5 main groups of rule changes. These changes include; the height of the net; court dimensions; service block/attack; buttocks determining plays; and, the joust and penetration. In many other cases of rule changes, Sitting Volleyball has accepted the indoor volleyball rule changes trends. Since Sitting Volleyball has been codified, the indoor game has gone through some drastic changes, including the way the game is scored, from scoring only from service to rally point, the number of points won to win a set, from 15points to 25 points and always 2 clear points difference in score. Other changes include the service zone covering the entire base line, back row line extensions and coach free zone, inclusion of technical time outs, and the introduction of liberos into team compositions. Sitting Volleyball tried to adopt the standing volleyball point's classification system that included team composition classification points were not allowed to exceed a certain number, but it was quickly abolished to a simpler classification system of disabled and minimally disabled. There could be revisions of the disability classification in the sitting game in the near future.

Some of the most complex rules include the lifting of the body when playing the ball and how technology may end up having some influence on refereeing decisions. More and more competitions are able to use hi-quality videoing systems to help with action replay. Competition organisers may have to consider how the use of 'challenges' by teams may impact the flow and interrupt the game. The ultimate way for people to understand what was the decision of the referee is to be able to understand the signals of the referees. The diagrams that determine the referee interpretations can be found in the official rule books of Sitting Volleyball. Although it should also be noted, that referees currently use a system whereby they sequence their calls and decisions. At first the referee blows the whistle. This commences serve, of which the referee will signal appropriately. The next time the referee blows a whistle is to end the rally. Then they indicate which team wins the point. After they have indicated this, they will provide another signal, indicating why they have won the point. To be able to follow the game without too much confusion, both the first and second referee will resort to mirroring each other's signal. After watching the rally, see how the referee produces a signal to see what had happened and why one team scored and not the other.

SECTION 2
Playing the Game

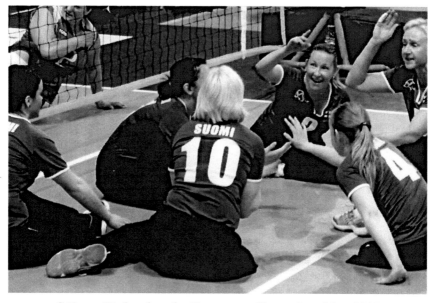

© Team Finland at the European Championships 2009

5 TEAM SYSTEMS

The reception component of the game is often considered the most important aspect of playing volleyball. Without a good service reception, it is easier for the opponents to score a point. Historically, when points were won only on a point-on-serve format, a weak reception often created a huge advantage for the serving team, as they could win the game with ease. The effect from a weaker reception is that it makes it harder for the setter to generate a good set, and therefore, makes it harder for the attacker to score from the first phase. Often, a poor reception will mean that the setter does not have all the options available to distribute to, and therefore it is easier to defend against the most likely attacker. This then, makes the modern game of volleyball an exciting game, as teams have placed a lot more concentration on the abilities of defence. Irrespective of who serves the ball, every serve leads to scoring or losing a point, which makes these two components of the game; reception and defence, important for team success.

Despite the changes in the nature of point scoring in volleyball, Sitting Volleyball also followed suit in 2000, and the focus on service reception is still regarded as an important component to the game. The individual skills for the execution of service reception have also changed in the modern game. The ball can be played without being called a technical fault with upper hands as well as with underarms. This is an important change in the way the game is played and it also affects the position of the reception unit.

When the ball could only be played with underarms, the ball is rebounded from the lower proportion of the body. In standing volleyball, that is basically anything under the height of the waist downwards. Most standing players have a spatial range of 1metre below the waist which they can reach and play with. In Sitting Volleyball, the range for playing an underarm movement is much less. In standing volleyball as well as playing the ball underarm, and the upper torso of a player can be reached in the range of also 1 metre. At least half of the balls played at the height of the upper torso are played with an overarm pass. The biomechanics of the player do not permit overhand passes from below chest level. Mechanically, in order to play the ball, the palms are turned upwards, and thus turning the shot into an underarm pass. However, the ability of being able to play the ball with the palms up at all heights can only be utilised when the trajectory of the ball is appropriate to go towards the desired target, and not going behind the head. Prevention of playing the ball backwards is made by turning the wrists (pronation) so that an overarm pass can be played.

Indoor volleyball players, not only have the freedom to move their legs, as they stabilise their platform for the receiving pass, they also have more time and more range of movement to play an appropriate and a good quality shot. Sitting Volleyball uses the dual function of the hands, for both movement assistance and playing the ball. Similar to football, whereby the player moves with their feet and has to find some balance to kick the ball with their feet, Sitting Volleyball athletes have been able to show exceptional skills and talent by using their hands and rebounding the ball to their desired place.

The use of the hands in moving and playing generates a significant time pressure to be in the right place, to choose the right type of shot to play, and to play the shot with quality.

High reactive speeds of the player to play a good pass are needed. Not only do they have to decide what type of pass they'll have to make, they need to move in place to play that ball optimally. In order to increase the chances of a good reception, the placement of the players, in relation to the server is important.

With the court being shorter, and the net lower, the receiving unit can often display a variety of court positions. These positions are dependent upon the attacking format, the rotation and position of the players, the strengths and weaknesses of the reception unit, and where the service blockers are.

The overhand reception has become far more common in the sitting game in recent times because of the issues raised; distance to play the ball in relation to the body; smaller court, lower net; dual use of arms for moving and playing; and starting position of the reception unit.

This chapter looks at the role of two specialist players that are heavily influential in the reception systems, namely the Libero and the setter. However, it starts with a section on a unique characteristic of Sitting Volleyball; the service block.

5.1 Service blocking

During the 1960s, the service block was removed from the indoor game. However, in Sitting Volleyball, the service block is a fundamental rule that can ultimately affect the tactics and systems used for receiving the opponents serve. By creating a block of the service, teams try to protect part of the court from the power serve. Thus making it easier for the reception to formulate an attack, as this gives a good receiving ball for the setter. Like in most situations, the blocker can either set themselves up to block the ball, or they can set themselves up to defend a part of the court.

For the service block, blockers that attempt to block the ball, tell the receivers which part of the court to cover. The position of the blocker tends to be placed in the main direction of the power serve. Serves that have too much power will go out of the court if the trajectory is too high, and the purpose of this block is to prevent low balls that go over the net entering that part of the court. This gives the server a choice to either serve the ball to a specific part of the court, where there will be a receiver to pick up the ball or with less power and higher trajectory aim to go over the block. The latter option usually gives the receiver enough time to move for the slower ball that goes over the block so that the team can form an attack.

Service blocking can also be used to cover a part of the court. Unsimilar to blocking the power serve, the position of the blocker is determined by the receivers. The receiving team tells where the blocker should be positioned so that it is possible for the team to set up an attack. This is more common when movement of players to go into position for the attack is an important part of the team tactics.

The service block can be reduced to one or two players depending on the situation. An advantage of having one less blocker is to have more receivers. More receivers of the serve mean more people can that cover the court. Another advantage of using fewer blockers is to position players so they are ready to formulate an attack.

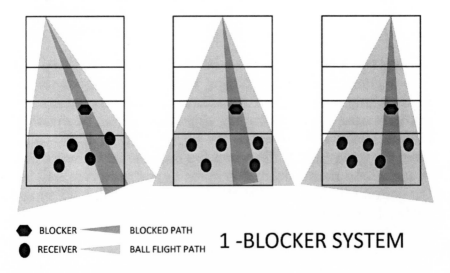

BLOCKER — BLOCKED PATH
RECEIVER — BALL FLIGHT PATH

1 -BLOCKER SYSTEM

12. 1 Blocker (W+1) format

The diagram in figure 12 demonstrates the blocked trajectory of the common one blocker systems from three typical areas of serve. Since players can serve from anywhere along the service line, the receiving unit and blocker needs to adjust itself accordingly. The darkened parts are areas that the blockers aim to cover or *"zone out"*. It does not mean the servers cannot serve to that part of the court, but it will mean that the server will serve with less power or with a higher trajectory to fall inside. The lightly shaded parts are potential areas for the serve to hit with power.

In all diagrams, the teams will place a player with good service reception skills in those parts of the court left by the blocker. When the opponents serve cannot be blocked because the trajectory is upward and over the block, sometimes the blocker will remove themselves from the block and help with the reception. There may be other cases, where the player is better at receiving than blocking and the team is better off with less blocking players.

In all cases, teams must evaluate their own strengths and weaknesses when deciding which system to adopt throughout the game, or for just for certain rotations and set pieces. Positions of players on the court can determine how much are their chances in winning a point against the service, in other words, to side-out. A typical 2 player block system is shown in figure 13.

Another way to form the reception unit is to put up two blockers and position the other four players on the court as receivers. In most cases, the four players will form an arc so that they cover the space that balls go over, as well as around the block. With this effective strategy, the one of the four receivers can be a front court player, and will have enough time to approach the net for an open set that is high and wide. One of the two blockers is in a good position to play the quick middle attack, or if the middle player is the setter, the attacker can move off from the net and approach for a ball set towards them. By using two blockers, teams which can cover a lot of the court with three receiving players, will often use the extra player as the reception target. This player is often treated as

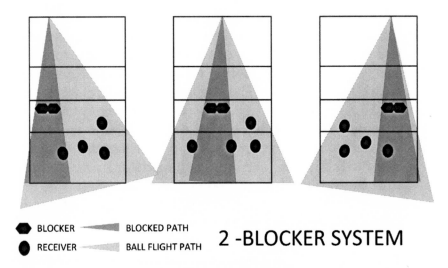

⬡ BLOCKER ◀━━ BLOCKED PATH
● RECEIVER ◀━━ BALL FLIGHT PATH

2 -BLOCKER SYSTEM

13. 2 Blockers reception

the setter as they will look to set the ball for the front court players. By disguising the setter, the opposition will have to spend more time and resources in deciphering the intentions of the attack so they can defend the ball. More about the service block and setter systems are in the latter sections on setting and backrow setting formations.

The final variation of how to put the blockers is to have all three frontrow players at the net to form a block. There are three main types of systems here. The most basic is to put three blockers collectively (see figure 14). Their function is to reduce the zone of the court and place the best receivers in parts of the court that are not covered by the block. Placement of the block is based on the ability of the server, with the intention to make the server play the ball from another part of the service line, or to play the ball where there is less power or control.

An alternative way to collective blocking is to place two blockers together and the third blocker by itself (see figure 15). By splitting the court, the server has a specific area to aim at so to avoid the block. The single blocker needs to be effective, and the reception unit has to be ready for a variety of serves include short serves that the blockers cannot reach.

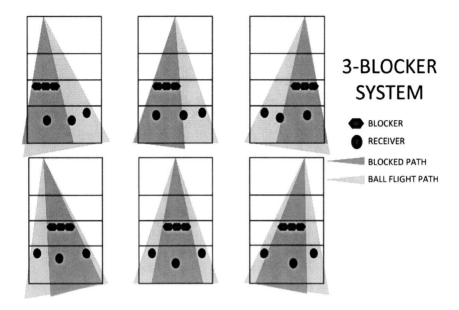

14. 3 Blockers collective

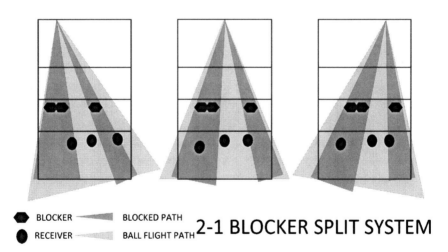

15. 2-1 Blockers split

The way the blockers are split can differ depending on the front line, position of setter and direction of serve. A blocking formation would use a 2-1 split, while an attacking formation with the setter in position 2 or 3 will use a 1-2 split (see figure 16). Using 3 lots of single blockers can also be effective in reducing the court for the receivers' positions.

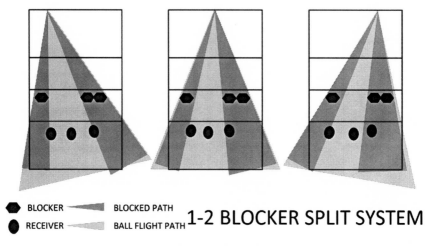

BLOCKER ◆ ▬▬▬ BLOCKED PATH
RECEIVER ● ▬▬▬ BALL FLIGHT PATH **1-2 BLOCKER SPLIT SYSTEM**

16. 1-2 Blocker Split system

5.2 Position of receivers

The position of the receivers is important as teams look to cover the court successfully. Doing this well will give the team a better chance to make an effective attacking play, so to score against the serving team. This is known as sideout in volleyball. The same applies to Sitting Volleyball, although there might be difficulties in the number of combinations setters have, which can make it harder for the team to sideout.

In all volleyball games, a well worked sequence from receive to set to attack is important when having to score enough points to win a set. In Sitting Volleyball, the attacker has much of the court coverage taken away by the block than the percentage of court available in standing volleyball. In top level standing volleyball, the attacker has a higher spiking contact point than their blocking counterpart. Tests have shown the spike approach generates higher vertical reach than a block jump. Since Sitting Volleyball is played sitting down, this difference does not seem so apparent. Some attackers may actually find their spike contact point is lower than the opposing blocker and there is very little the athlete can do to overcome this. Standing players can train their jumping abilities, while sitting players have to adopt various attacking styles against different types of blockers.

Other ways to help the attackers is to position the receivers in a way to cover a part of the court, whereby the attackers has the strongest advantage to go against a weak block. Therefore, the position of the receivers and the front court players will depend on the ability of the players and their position on the court. Coverage of the court can be reduced by the proportion of the court covered by the service block. Although the blockers do not eliminate the zone completely, the function of the block is to prevent the penetration of the most powerful serve, and if the ball was to go over the block, it would be less powerful and thus, a player would have sufficient time to react to the ball. The reaction can lead to minor movement that is needed to play the ball well enough so that the ball can be used by other team mates.

The fundamental rule of the receiving team is to distribute the court between the receivers. The use of the Libero can often make a stronger reception unit. If the players are of equal ability and the court is divided fairly, each player would be responsible of 2m wide x 2.5m length court space. Players need to know how they can cover this part of the court, and where any overlapping between players can be achieved without injuring the other teammate. There are then exceptions where a person with more mobility may take responsibility of more space and a person with less mobility takes less space. Often the ability to move laterally is harder than being able to move backwards. Since the rules allowed the use of the forehands on the service reception, the receivers can start their receiving position closer to the net. In this way, although the player is closer to the ball, the players have a sense of distortion by receiving the ball from closer than further away. The first reason for doing this is to reduce the angle of serve. The same strategy is used in tennis on a regular basis. When the players approach the net, they reduce the angle from which the player can pass the ball on the court. The player at the net does not need to travel as far as the angle is less. It also forces the opponent to play in other parts of the court, often causing risks and subsequently errors. In tennis, players who do not feel comfortable in playing a shot past the net player will go for the lob shot. This gives them time to recover, and if the lob isn't too high, but is deep enough, it'll force the player to the back of the court. Sitting Volleyball servers will also have to face similiar issues too. The receiving team can also create a faster attack, although time is virtually eliminated when the reception plays a high ball towards the setter. However, if the ball is played quickly back into the opponent's court, it can catch the serving team by surprise

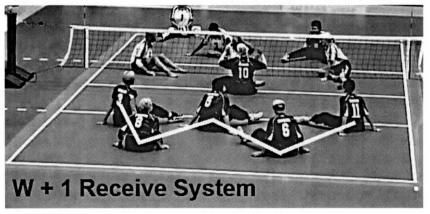

W + 1 Receive System

17. Photograph of W+1 system

and place them under pressure or make it unreachable.

As in the indoor game, there are basic formations for the reception unit in Sitting Volleyball. However, these formations can, if necessary, include the service block. A basic volleyball formation is the W+1 system. Only one player at the net is blocking, and the other 5 players form a 'W' shape on the court. The axis of the 'W' shape is dependent on position from where the server is. Ideally, the 'W' should be facing the server, so the distance between the server and the back two receivers are of equal distance. In this formation, the players have less width to cover, and since moving laterally is often harder than moving backwards, this system is a good base for a team to cover the court and reduce the amount of aces a server can make.

The main problem that comes from this system is that it has only one service blocker. This gives many more angles of the court for the server to aim at. The blocker might also be the setter, and if they are positioned towards the left of the court, the blocker will then have to turn and move to position 2 to set the ball. Since the other two front court players are part of the reception formation, they will have to transition from receive to attack, and this almost eliminates the possibility of a quick middle attack. Despite these problems, teams still like to utilise this type of system as it is a safe way to reduce the amount of service aces. For teams with less mobility, players can move more easily forwards and backwards without having to worry much about moving side to side. The players can also hit the ball away from the net, and the attack is done intelligently, where they can reduce the chances of getting blocked.

5.3 **Libero**

The word, 'Libero' comes from the Italian word for 'free'. It was eventually accepted as a position in volleyball whereby a player can change for any other backrow player without the necessity of an official substitution. The players were free to move in and out of court, once in the backrow. The Libero can be easily identified on the court, because the colour of the jersey is different from the other players. Liberos were introduced to the game of volleyball in 1998. Since then, there have been several changes in the Libero rule around the world. Teams can now have two Liberos in their squad, however only one of them can be on court at any one time. Other restrictions of the Libero player comes from the philosophy that the player must be good defender, and therefore, Liberos are not allowed to serve the ball into the court, and they must not make an attack when the entire ball is higher than the top of the net. When the team rotates to a position whereby the libero is supposed to go to the front court, then the player they replaced has to come back onto the court.

In the indoor game, the use of a Libero can help strengthen the attack as the player is a specialist that only takes the ball from service or is positioned in a place to defend the ball. It also gives the player he/she replaces a chance to have a bit of a break from the power exertion from jumping, landing, hitting, and blocking while playing at the net. However, in Sitting Volleyball, players in the front court cannot leave the ground due to the 'lifting' rule. The teams can often rely more on the back court attacker in the sitting game than standing, and it may therefore mean that teams do not need to use a libero all of the time.

Depending on the team composition, teams that use a libero will find two players with whom the Libero can exchange. The easiest to manage is when the two players are opposite each other. In the indoor game, it is often the middle blockers that the libero will exchange with. While in the sitting game, the position of the player that goes off can depend more on the player's disability rather than their front court playing position. For example, a player may have a very powerful hitting action, but has only one arm. In this case, they would be very useful to play in the attacking zone. Once in the backrow, the Libero that has two arms can be more useful as more space of the court can be easily defended. A player that has more mobility might also be at an advantage over a player who is slow in moving around the backcourt.

The exchange of a MD player might also help facilitate the regular substitution of another MD player into another part of the court. If the MD player is in the backcourt, the coach may take that MD off the court and at the same time, have the other MD player approach the substitution zone. Now that the Libero has taken the place of the MD player, the team is without an MD until the substitution is complete. If the substituted player was opposite the original MD player, then the team has three rotations to benefit from having an MD in the front court. When the Libero is forced to come back off the court, since positioned in the front court, the original MD player goes to the frontrow and the other MD moves to position 1 and is expected to serve the ball. The coach now has a decision as to whether the new MD should be substituted off, or if the team works better with the new MD, even though the MD is in the backrow. Following this choice, coaches will make another substitution so that only one MD is on the court at any time.

Liberos do not have to be constantly on the court. Even if they appear on the score sheet, their involvement might not be needed. Teams may decide to not use the Libero for the entire game, but in another match, find them having to use the Libero as often as possible. Some teams only use the Libero by replacing just one player throughout the entire match. The other 5 players continue to play in their positions or are substituted off in a regular way.

The use of the Libero in the reception unit can be very beneficial for the team. Since the Libero player is one of the best defence players, if not the best player on the team, they will also have the responsibility to replace a player that has poor skills in receiving. The service reception is a very important aspect in terms of building up an attack. Conversely, the opponents are using the serve as a weapon and a means to score a direct point. Therefore, in order to counter the power of serves and reduce the intention to score a point, teams can train a player to specially deal with this problem and this specialist can also be the Libero.

Since players can serve from anywhere along the backline, the direction of the incoming ball can vary a lot. Players in the front line can set up the service block so that any tough serves need to go around or over the block. Typically, teams will want to make the server aim and play the ball towards the Libero, in that way, it is easier for the receiving team to build up an attack. Some occasions this is very difficult to achieve because the server can still penetrate parts of the court whereby the block has not covered and there is no Libero there. In these situations, the team's line-up needs to be fixed whereby the receiver has strong enough skills to make a sufficient pass. It may also mean that the coach needs to make a substitution of receiving players as the Libero is not used.

The introduction of the Libero system makes team dynamics lively and is a creative element in the game. As well, since these players are defence specialists, it should mean the duration of the rallies are longer as the ball is controlled better than other players. Subsequently, with better ball control, the setter has more options to set the ball, and the attacker can have an easier time to hit the ball with power. All in all, with better defence, there are better attacks, which push the players to defend better, and the cycle goes on.

5.4 Setting

There are a number of team systems that are based on the number of setters and attackers. The more advanced the players are, the more complex the team system can become, leading to opponents experiencing difficulties to respond. At the most basic level, teams will often find it difficult to aim the ball towards a certain part of the court for a player to set. The most important thing is to stop the server from scoring an ace. After being successful in getting the ball up, the ball must travel high enough for another player to safely set the ball for a player to attack. This is basic three touch volleyball. There are many disadvantages to this system too. If the ball is set from a backrow player, the spiker has to look at the ball that is coming from over their shoulder to attack the ball. If the ball comes from either their side, or in front of them, then the spiker can also see where the blockers and defenders are on the opponent's court. Rather than looking at the ball coming from over their shoulder, it is easier to place balls into the opponent's court when the player has the ball in front of them. The player that sets the ball needs to communicate with other players to inform them that they will be setting the ball. In this way, the player may find that they might lose a fraction of a second to make the decision of whether it is a ball that is within reach to set, or if another player is in a better position. After going through this evaluation, the ball may have dropped lower and would be in a difficult position to set. The more time it takes for the team players to decide who sets the ball, the more the risk the team has in being able to produce a good set, and score.

5.4.1 **Position 3**

Often teams try to make a systematic way of positioning the setter. If the receivers have a target to aim at, the most straight forwards way is to play the ball to position 3. Teams will find that it is easier to reduce the time it takes to make the decision of whether another player should play the ball or not, if the ball goes to position 3. The player in position three is therefore the designated setter for the team, in that rotation. When the team rotates, a new player takes up position 3 and becomes the setter. This is a simple and effective way of creating a system. The problem with this is that the ball will often come from behind the setter at position 3. This makes it harder for the setter to see where the opponent's block is being based before they make a decision of where to play the ball to. Just as with the Libero position, the setter requires specialist training. If a player is not very good at setting the ball along the net for their team-mate to spike, then it is likely the team would struggle when that player is in position 3.

A solution to the problem of setting from any player in position 3, is to have a better player to set the ball. Other than making a tactical substitution, as the team's ball control gets better, they will start to evaluate how to get the ball to a player who is in the best position to set the ball. Many teams will change their setting position to either position 2 or position 3. If there is a player in position 3 and they need vast improvement in their skill levels, then teams can do one of the two following things. They could move the players along the net, thus keeping the same target area for the receivers to aim at. The movement of players will mean another player has temporarily switched places so that a different player with setting skills is in position 3. The player originally in position 3, who moved out the way, is now going to become a spiker in the position from where they have momentarily switched with the setter. Alternatively, the spiker becomes an extra attacker along the front row. This composition is usually seen by high level teams, and there can be specific systems for creating more front row attackers. However, to continue with the development of role of the setter, the other option is to make the players play the ball to another position instead of position 3.

5.4.2 Setting the ball from position 2

In most cases, playing the ball to position 2 is highly beneficial. This is usually because setters have a better angle from which the ball comes in from, they can see the position of the attackers on their own side of the court, as well as sensing the whereabouts the opponents and how they are positioned on the other side of the net. Moreover, when the ball comes from position 2, if the spikers are right handed, then the ball can be attacked at various tempos, heights and with a lot of accuracy. The attackers are also at an advantage, because as the ball is being hit, the spiker can see the ball, the opposition's blocking unit and defenders. Everything is in front of them. Also, since the ball is coming towards them, it is easier to make good ball control with the hand than it is to hit the ball from behind the shoulder, whereby the ball's trajectory is already going over the net. By positioning the setter in position two, the middle attack can play the quick attack. A constant threat comes from the attacker in the middle of the court as the ball is literally snatched from the setter. Depending on the distance away from the setter and the middle attacker, there are the possibilities that the attacker actually plays the second ball over the net without the setter touching the ball. This strategy is usually effective when the opposite blockers are waiting for the setter to make a decision.

Teams may also decide to play the ball to position 4. This is a good strategy in Sitting Volleyball, because most players are right handed. If the ball is well controlled, then it may pose a threat to the opponents as the ball is ready to be hit instead of set. By making this threat, teams will have to start blocking in position 4, which leaves more holes along the net for the other two front court attackers to hit from. To give the attacker holes to hit into, the player in position 4 has to decide to set the ball instead of spiking it. Teams may also do this because they have left handed players in the front court. Having players that can spike with their left hand can greatly improve the dynamic nature of a team's offense. Setting the ball in position 4, to players who hit with their left hand has, in principle, the same advantages as a right-handed spiker hitting a ball from position 2.

5.4.3 Triangle system

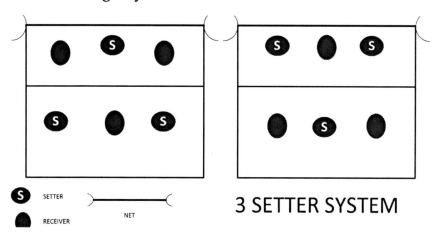

3 SETTER SYSTEM

18. 3 Setter Systems

If teams want to start specialising the role of players, a simple way to do this is to play a triangle setting system. In this system, every other player on the court is the setter and the setter in the front court can either be in position 2, 3, or 4. On some occasions there will be two setters on the front court, and this can cause many problems to the opponents when trying to work out who is going to set the ball. To complicate things further, all six players are potential attackers. When there is only one setter, that setter is in position 3. Teams then have the option to either set from that position 3 or the setter moves to position 2 and the other player in position 2 goes to spike in the middle.

The movement of players along the net for a receiving team that has a service block is not the easiest of tasks to do, however it can be a rather effective way of generating attacks. Teams that practice well the service reception rotations can often find good solutions to problems and create combinations of attacks as well as a variety of attacks that will surprise the opposition and are spectacular for the audience to see.

5.4.4 **Four setters**

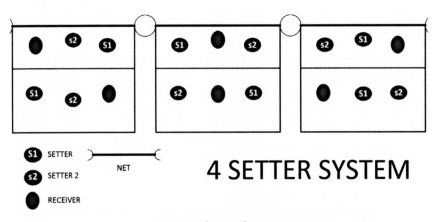

4 SETTER SYSTEM

19. 4:2:2 Setter System

Teams with less mobility may opt for a system whereby there are four setters. This system tends to operate with two primary and two secondary setters. The primary setters are opposite each other and the secondary setters are also opposite each other. This leaves the non-setters opposite each other. When the primary setters are in either position 2 or 3, they will set the ball. Only when the primary setter is in position 4, will the secondary setter take on the main setting responsibilities. If the main target for the receivers is position two, then the main setter will rotate in front of the secondary setter. That is, if the primary setter is in position 2, then the secondary setter is in position 3. This way, when the primary setter goes to serve, the other primary setter is in position 4 and the secondary setter is in position 2. The receiving unit will then aim to get the ball to position 2. The order of the setters will change if the main target for the receivers is position 3. This means only 2 of the 6 rotations will the setter be in position 2, while the other 4 rotations, a setter will be in position 3.

The utilisation of four setters requires balance in the team and operates best when most of the players' have all rounded skills. They will each have the responsibility to receive and attack. Only two of the players will not be required to set the ball, and players with the responsibilities are opposite each other. It is a straight forward system that can enable structured Libero changes, depending on the attributes of a team and the position of the servers. Since teams are not so mobile, when the setter is in position three, it is the only time where they can set the ball to right side attacker. As opposed to setting the ball to the middle and left side of the court, dealing with right sided attacks is another consideration for a defensive unit.

5.4.5 Four attackers and two setters

If people were asked what the favourite thing to do in volleyball is, most people would say they like to hit the ball. It is the shot that can visibly score points, and is the most frequent way to score. It could also be said that it is the most complex shot to make and therefore a lot of practice goes into it. Teams may find that they have more spikers than setters and it becomes useful for them to have a two setter system and the other players become spikers. The two setters are positioned opposite each other so that there is always a setter in the front court or backcourt. The other four spikers become general spikers, with some having preferences to attack at different parts of the net, while others attack anywhere along the net.

Due to the rotation nature of the game, the use of a two setter system will encourage movement between players. There will be at least two rotations where the setter will move from the base position to the setter's position. In most cases, there is the movement to position two or three. There are two common ways of making this movement. The most popular route is for the setter in position 1 to move to position 2 (see figure 20).

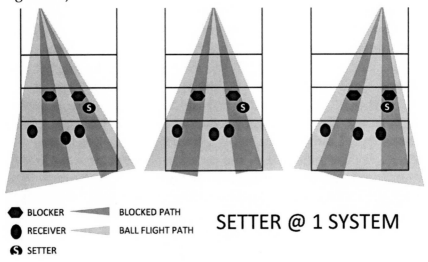

BLOCKER — BLOCKED PATH

RECEIVER — BALL FLIGHT PATH

SETTER

SETTER @ 1 SYSTEM

20. Setter at Position 1

This way, the teams will have three attackers along the net for that rotation. The setter in position 4 acts as a spiker in this rotation. Advancements to this system are to move the setter from position 6 up to position 2, as this will also create 3 front row attackers (see figures 21 and 22).

When the setter is in position 5, it is very difficult to move across the court, and in this way, the setter in position 2 can take the responsibility to distribute the ball to the other two front court attackers or to play a back court set.

The setters have a lot of responsibility to ensure they will play the second contact. In some cases, if the reception is of poor quality, the setter will have to resort to chasing the ball and then have to play the ball under pressure. Often the advantages of having a third front court attacker is far greater than the threat of a second ball coming over the net, and in this way, teams will strive for this. At other times, the setter in position 4 can continue to threaten the opponents

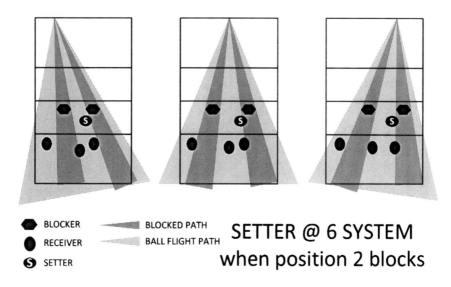

BLOCKER   BLOCKED PATH
RECEIVER   BALL FLIGHT PATH
SETTER

SETTER @ 6 SYSTEM
when position 2 blocks

21. Setter at Position 6 when blocker is at 2

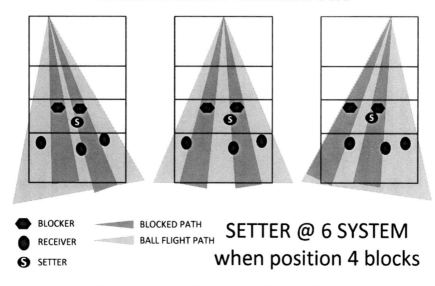

BLOCKER   BLOCKED PATH
RECEIVER   BALL FLIGHT PATH
SETTER

SETTER @ 6 SYSTEM
when position 4 blocks

22. Setter at Position 6 when blocker is at 4

by attacking a second ball instead of setting it to an attacker. If blockers cannot move very well, then it might be more sensible to play the ball to where ever the setter is positioned, so that an effective attack can be formed.

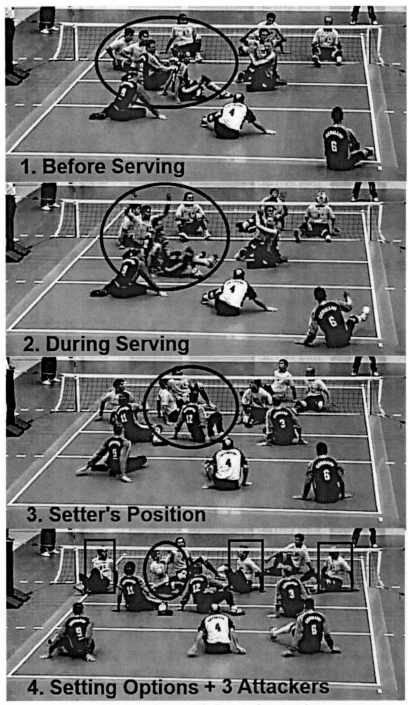

23. Movement of players for attack

Other times, teams may want to play the ball to only position 2 and 3. This is because it can be quite confusing for the receiving player to direct their pass to different parts of the court. Without much practice or especially, when they are put under immense pressure during the game, direction of the ball might be less than optimal. As a receiving unit, the spiker prefers to move away from the net before moving forward in their spike approach. If the receiver sends the ball to position 2, but the setter is in position 4, then it will mean the spiker will have to change the momentum of movement and instead of attacking the ball, might have to rescue it, and if lucky, another team player has enough time to spike the ball. On the other hand, if the setter who is in position 4 has moved to position 3, then the ball goes to position 2, the setter is already moving and can chase the ball so that the ball can be set, even to the right side attacker.

This last example might only be used by teams when one of the setters is in the front court. It is used by teams that have one dominant setter and the opposite player to the setter only sets the ball when the setter is in position 5. Playing a one setter system is incredibly difficult in the sitting game. The setter must be mobile and the team needs to have a lot of strategic attacking combinations to make it worthwhile for teams to execute. The ability to play a one setter system also depends on the opponents serve and how effective the service blocking unit is. A setter who has to block in position 4 and then move to position 2 to set the ball will need a nice and easy high ball from the receiver. Meanwhile the accompanying service blocker in position 3 will have to move to a position so that they are ready to spike the ball with full force and accuracy before the setter can set the ball. To make it easier, the service block might be positioned closer to the centre of the court, which will leave the line open for the server to play the ball to. A strong serve down the line is often a hard ball for the receiver to control, and it may mean that the setter has to move to another part of the court to set the ball anyway. In order to help the receiver, either a Libero can take the line ball, place two receivers in this area, or the last option would be to move the block to cover the line, and the setter having more distance to travel if s/he is going to set from position 2 or 3.

5.5 **Summary**

The reception unit is an integral part of a winning team. Teams that have good strategies against a variety of serves will find it easier to play their game. Teams that fail upon the pressure of an opponent's serve can collapse as they struggle to find a solution to overcome the serves. When this happens, the coach has three main options;

◘ to change the receiving unit's position;
◘ to change players;
◘ to call a time-out and try to disrupt the flow of the opposition's server.

All teams can hope for the server to make a mistake, but this gives up control to the opponent and not of your own team. Team tactics depend on a variety of variables, some that are within the control of the team, and some that are controlled by the serving team. Lining up against the opponent's strengths and weakness is a necessity when choosing how the reception unit can prevail under the pressure of the opponent's serve. The reception unit will need to consider the following;

◘ the position of the court from which the server serves from
◘ the rotation of the receiving team and the setter system used
◘ the placement of the Libero in each of the rotations
◘ the opponent's blocking rotation

6 DEFENSIVE SYSTEMS

Defence is an important component of winning volleyball. Getting a defensive system correct can make the difference between winning and losing. Although many coaches will spend a lot of time on transition play and the attack, most would also agree that spending a good amount of practice time on defensive strategies pays off. In fundamental terms, the attacker has around 70-85% chance of scoring against the defender. The easiest way the attacker can get a point is when the opponent makes a technical mistake, such as a net touch or invasion under the net. In Sitting Volleyball, the buttocks determine the position of the player and whether penetration into the opponent's court has occurred. It is therefore very difficult to invade under the net and into the opponent's court. It is not the same as indoor volleyball and forcing opponents to make such an error is often not possible. Forcing a net touch might be a little more feasible though. If the defence does not force a net violation, then the attacker can score points in a number of other ways; block-out; block-in, spike kill, tip kill, or, defensive error.

Hitting a block-out is based on a very technical ability to hit the hands or fingers of the blocker in a way whereby the ball comes off the block and lands out of court. To score a block-in point, players force the ball past the block whereby the ball lands on the blockers side of the court. This requires a bit of luck and a lot of power in the swing to make sure the blocked shot does not go back over the net to the attacker's side. A spike kill is the most obvious way of scoring, and there are high percentages of these points when there is a poorly designed defensive system. If all the players and the block give a part of the court whereby there is no one there, it is the spiker's pleasure to hit that part of the court to score a point with power and accuracy. A tip kill is a useful means of scoring a point when the attacker sees a gap in the defence and can place the ball to that part of the court, either with the fingertips, or rolling the ball. Attackers can also force defensive errors too. When the defence is in a rush, the attacker can play the ball towards the player, whereby they cannot control the ball and the ball goes out of play, or it goes back over the net but lands out. Shots like these require high levels of teamwork that go against the defensive system.

With all these ways to score a point, the percentage of scoring always favours the attacking team. Many teams will spend a lot of time perfecting their attack as this is what helps them score points. However, there will also be many occasions where the opportunity to score is reduced considerably due to the way the defensive system is set up.

6.1 **Fundamentals of Defence**

The ball is hit from at least 1.05m or 1.15m off the ground, and it has to land within 5 metres of the net. This angle of descent is much less than hitting from 2.24m or 2.43m from the ground to land within 9m. That is to say, in the indoor game, the maximum distance (from the top of the net) an attacker has to hit the ball is 12.96m or 12.92m (for women). In the beach game, the court is one metre shorter, so the maximum distance is 11.57m or 11.53m (for women). The maximum distance for Sitting Volleyball court is 7.89m or 7.88m (for women). Test results from the velocity of a spiked ball averaged at 30metres per second. Using these speeds, indoor volleyball spikes takes 0.57 seconds for the ball to hit the furthest distance. In Sitting Volleyball the time is reduced to 0.34 seconds.

Track (athletics) sprinters' reactions are somewhere between 0.14 and 0.16 seconds. However, this type of reaction leads to only one type of response, and that is to run. They rely on the use of sound from the starting gun and do not need to take into account other external and distracting variables. Volleyball players rely on the visual aspect of the game, and there are a multitude of movements that are required. It therefore slows down the neurological processes to react and these human reaction times will be slower than sprinters.

Tests on athletes' reaction times based on decision making have recorded results in the range of 0.20-0.40seconds. These results were based on laboratory settings and determined repetitive movement types after a given stimulus. To translate this information for volleyball specifics, some slight discrepancies are needed and there are claims that 0.30-0.40 seconds is a reasonable statement, but it might be worthwhile to have this number range widened to 0.20-0.40seconds.

When players also have to move, by using their hands, they may not have any time at all to play the ball with accuracy, and instead learn to use their entire body to rebound the ball up into the air. As such, to have successful defence, the positioning of the players is of the utmost importance.

6.2 Blocking

Blocking in Sitting Volleyball has the same purposes as in indoor volleyball. These are to score a point from the opponent's attack, to return the ball to the opponent's court, to slow down the attacker's shot, or make the attacker to hit towards another part of the court. The sitting game also permits the use of the service block, which has the same purposes as in a defensive block. During the game, the defensive block is used against attackers. Teams have up to three touches to formulate an attack, and in Sitting Volleyball, any one of the three shots can be a potential threat. In this way, the block needs to be alert from the opponent's first contact. Blockers need to also be ready for the second ball over, before finally preparing for a third touch attack.

6.2.1 **Base positions**

All the front row players are capable of blocking the opponent. Teams may have a number of blocking systems, and this can often determine the base positions of the block. In other situations, the block base position can be determined by the match up of attacker and blocker, and the position of the setter. Placing the strongest blocker against the strongest attacker can reduce the impact from the attacking team, and improve defensive strategies. Teams that are confident in defence may end up arranging their players so they are ready for attack. The main component for an attack is to have the setter in an optimal position. If this is in position two, the setter will be designated to hold the block position.

In a one-on-one situation, the blocker is up against the attacker, and has to readjust the block according to the direction of the attacker or the type of shot that the attacker plays. The base of the block is dependent on the probability of the attacker's approach to play a ball at a certain part along the net. In the majority of cases, lining up the block with the attacker's main swing is effective for defence. Talented attackers, who can cut and swipe attacks with accuracy and power will find it easier to hit against such a block. To reduce the impact of the attacker, teams might want to put a collective block along the net.

In order to make a collective block, the base position of the middle blocker is to be close to the middle of the court, whereby the blocker will be able to close the block, set by the outside blockers using little effort. In general, closing the block is when the hands of the blockers are sealed so that a ball cannot travel between them. The outside blockers base position will be around a metre away from the antenna so that the middle blocker has the flexibility to move as soon as they have the opportunity to go.

There are two main systems for blocking taken from the indoor game; read and react, and commit. The read and react block is based on the middle blocker waiting to see the setter's play before deciding which attacker to block. Once the ball has been set, the middle blocker chases after the ball and forms a collective block with the other team mate, the teammate that has set the outside of the block. The commit block is usually set up against faster attacks, and tends to leave a lot of one-on-one situations, although the most powerful attacks are stopped. It may mean that the middle blocker who is committed to blocking the middle player will not be actually blocking. If the ball is set to the outside, the middle blocker only has time to come off the net for a short distance to cover any balls that are tipped.

Whatever the system used for the situation, blockers will find that they are restricted from instantaneous blocking as they use their hands to push and pull themselves to the blocking position. Whereas, in the indoor game, the blocker may keep their hands up quite high and use their legs to get to the blocking position, the sitting player uses the hands for a dual purpose; to move and to play to the ball. If the hands are up in the air, the player will have very restricted movement around the court. In Sitting Volleyball, the correct base position is therefore important for an effective block.

The Sitting Volleyball blocker needs to move their hands at least a metre from the ground to be able to block the ball at the top of the net. To be able to move sufficiently, the player needs to push or pull their body with their hands. They then need to have their hands above their net to block the ball. If the average indoor volleyball player can touch the top of the net, then it is only a matter of centimetres to be able to reach above the net and block. Indoor volleyball blockers can use more time on accurate positioning of the block as well as covering more distance along the net. In the sitting game, the distance travelled from the ground to the top of the net to block is quite a lot. Hence, a combination of having an effective movement pattern from the base position, with fast hands to reach over the net is needed to combat the attack.

Most receiving teams will be positioned around 3metres from the net. The height of their hands to play an overhead volley pass as their chosen reception shot can be quite a lethal threat. Since the trajectory from an overhead volley pass can be flat as well as high, the receiver may decide to push the ball towards the opponents' court as an attacking shot. The blocker from the service team needs to be ready for this. In this case, the blocker who has just been part of block coverage from the service block has to be aware of the shortest line that the receiver would choose to make a direct attack. This type of shot is often seen from the receiver at the back left of the court and playing the ball to the back right of the serving team. This is mainly because, most servers who serve will end up defending the back right of the court, and this part of the court poses vulnerabilities. To prevent this, the front right blocker has to move from the service block coverage to the front right of the court and intercept any possibility of this shot. After the threat has gone by, either by the reception shot being sent to the setter or sent to another part of the court, the front right blocker can then adjust their base position for the attack. If the team receives the ball using an underhand pass, then the blocker can go from block coverage to their base position almost immediately. Underarm passes have an upward trajectory and it causes very little threat to the server

6.2.2 **Collective blocking**

Some of the issues of the indoor game for a collective block are; the timing of the blockers; the creation of a seam between the blockers; and, overall effect of the block on the attacker. Sitting Volleyball poses slightly different principles of collective blocking. Blockers are not jumping for height rather they just have to have their hands up. On the sitting court, the blockers use their hands to move first before raising their hands to block. The angle reduced by collective blocking is much more effective as there is less space for the attacker to hit the ball into. Bringing the block together to reduce the chance of a gap between the blockers still plays an important part in a collective block.

The middle blocker that is playing a read and react system needs to have long limbs to reach for the ball, and have a good pushing and pulling mechanisms to move sideways across the net. Blockers can set up their block early and not worry about the lowering of the block from a jump since they are sat on the floor. The timing of the block may not seem to be so important, but it is. Attackers that have a block that is put up too early may revert to using the block for a 'block-out' type of attack. They will also be able to use the existing block to readjust their attack so that can attack towards another part of the court. Blockers hands that are placed up high in the air may become useless as the attacker chooses to tip the ball rather than spike the ball. In these situations, the blockers that have set their position quickly for a slow attack will need to wait for their hands to reach over the net in time to form a block in relation with the attacker's swing. Then they need to finish the block for a block point.

3 blockers against an attacker is one of the hardest collective blocks to make. As well as the blocker having to travel almost the entire width of the court in time before the attacker swings at the ball, the defenders need to be aware of the remainder of the court that needs to be covered. The third blocker will need to be mindful of the attacking range, the blocking abilities of other teammates, and their own potential to transition from the position of blocking to retreat and formalise an attack with efficiency. Slow attacks in the middle, may find that three blockers are put up against the attacker, as the middle attacker has a range of shots to play and more angles to attack the ball than on other parts of the court. Although, in read and react systems, and the speed of middle attacks, it is also very difficult for blockers to be in position to block the middle and at the same time be far out enough to avoid collisions with the middle block that might end up going towards the antenna for a collective block.

6.2.3 **Jousting**

The blockers in the sitting game have to reach their hands over the net while their buttocks are still in contact with the ground. In this way, no loss of contact with the ground is permitted by the blocker's play. When this happens, the blockers have a stable base to play the ball. The advantage blockers then have is the use of the base to effectively block the ball. There is also consistency in the height of the block. When two players on both sides of the court go to block the ball at the net, they can find themselves pushing against each other with the ball. When the ball becomes stationary, they are 'jousting', and the point is replayed.

Although the joust rule had been pretty much eliminated in the indoor game, and has been completely removed from the beach game, the sitting game still uses the joust. The main reason for this is the fact that blockers are still in contact with the ground while blocking. This could mean that the held ball could be between two players for a very long time, as the block's height remains consistent. When this happens, no team is awarded a point, and the rally is replayed.

Jousting is a result of the blockers being in touch with the floor. Since players cannot jump and their block height varying due to jumping and landing, there can be a lot of action surrounding net. Blockers are allowed to block the ball and subsequently attack the ball. In the indoor game, blockers will find themselves waiting to land before playing the ball again. Since the blockers are already on the floor, the time between block and attack can be very short. The time it takes for players to convert from blocker to attack is much less and decision making between plays is reduced. Motor skill of the players at the net is very flexible. Balls between net players may go on several times without the player's hands ever touching the floor to move when the ball is being fought at the net. Once the hands fall below the top of the net, the opponent can have the advantage and score a point.

Blocking in the sitting game has the same principles as the indoor game, although its functions are vastly different due to time, speed of reactions, skills and position of players. Successful teams have realised the effectiveness of blocking and would have spent a lot of time in getting this component of the game working effectively. On an individual level, players are restricted in how they can improve the height of the block as they cannot jump to reach higher. Instead, they can work on improving their stability and the strength of their blocking base as well as fast reactions to motor movements for battles at the net.

6.3 Floor Defence

In Sitting Volleyball there are two common floor defensive systems used by international teams. A third system is often seen in developing women teams when the ability to move and covering the court is harder. The third system is often seen in club teams or masters' teams. These three popular systems come from the indoor volleyball game, but there are some minor modifications to cope with the angle of attack and the distance of the court. Popular systems depend on the block and the opponent's attacking power. The system that is the least demanding of the players movement is the flat line system. Players often find themselves in poor positions to play the ball, but can slow down the opponent's power. The most popular floor defensive systems used in Sitting Volleyball is from indoor volleyball called the '6-up defence', sometimes referred to as 'man-up defence'. While in indoor volleyball the most popular floor defensive system is the '6-back defence', or 'man-down', otherwise known as perimeter defence systems and is also used in the sitting game.

6.3.1 6-up system

The 6-up or sometimes known as the man-up defensive system is played with the defender at position 6 positioned behind the block. The other defenders are on the outer edges of the court, where they would be placed in an optimal position to defend the hard and fast driven spikes. The line defender is typically positioned somewhere between a metre and a 150cm from the back line and sitting comfortably just inside the line. The diagonal player is placed furthest away from the attacker and positions themselves approximately one metre in from the side line and one metre in from the end line. The non-blocking front row player comes off the net towards the 2 metre attack line. A typical 6-up defensive system can be seen in figure 24.

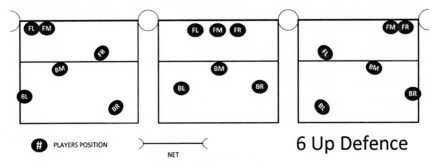

24. 6-up defence system

Using the 6-up defensive system has many benefits and these include;

- Positioning the backrow setter so that it can be easy to transition
- Covering behind the block for attacking tips
- Having a balanced defence against hard driven balls
- Useful with a big blocking team

There are also disadvantages to a 6-up defensive system;

- Leaves a big hole in the back court defence
- Can be dangerous for the 6-up defender when there is a hole in the block and the attacker hits directly to the 6-up defender
- May leave the 6-up defender too close to the net, in the front zone and the ball gets deflected back into the opponent's court. This is illegal if the entirety of the ball is above the net height at the point of contact with the defending player.

As it so happens, depending on the height of the defender, and their preferred way of defending, it may appear that the defender in position 1 is actually a lot closer to the net than it would be seen relation to an indoor volleyball court.

6.3.2 6-back system

The 6 defender stays back with the other two wing defenders starting up a bit in the 6-back or man-down defensive system. In this way, the defenders make a 'U' shaped defence. This places the player in position 6 in the best position to take a

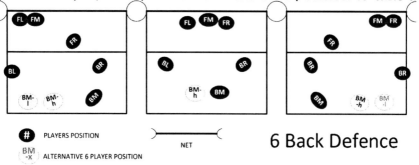

25. 6-back defence system

hard driven ball when there is a gap in the block, or from the passive block-out shot. Many attackers will hit into the top of the block so to achieve a block out against a set of over-reaching blockers. Depending on the blockers hands, it is very likely the ball will go from the top and deep outside of the court. In order for the defending team to rescue such an attack, the player in position 6 is deep in defence to tries and pick up the ball.

Meanwhile, since all the defenders go to the perimeter of the court, there are vulnerabilities just behind the block for the short tips or roll shots. Teams that use this system must be very certain that these short balls can also be recovered well enough for the next transition between defence and offense. Benefits from the 6-back defensive systems include;

- An player is in position to take attacks from a slow forming block that leaves a gap for the attacker
- If opponents go for high hand swipes, such as deep block-outs, the defence has a player ready to pick the balls that are falling out of the court.
- Tempts the attacker into making a tip or roll shot, whereby they make a mistake and can get blocked easily

Teams should also be weary of problems that 6-back defensive systems pose;

- Player in Position 6 will find it hard to get involved in the next transition from defence to offense
- A big hole forms for attackers to tip or roll the ball into behind the block and the middle of the court
- All balls that are played above the shoulders will be hit out, some players do not have time to move out of the way of an oncoming ball that is going out the court

There are also two more variations of the 6-back defence and that depends on the way the block is formed. If the blocker unit positions themselves to cover one part of the court, then the 6 defender will have to adjust their position to cover that part of the court that is left opened by the block. There are three typical ways, blocking line, blocking cross court and leaving the middle. When the blocking unit is blocking a line ball, the 6 defender (BM) goes towards the diagonal and joins the other diagonal defending player.

When the block is taking cross-court attacks, the 6 defender (BM-l) moves towards the other line defender and covers the line. It might mean the line defender is positioned up in defence to pick up the tips, and is ready to set the ball if it does not come to them. With this configuration, it is possible to overcome the problem of tip coverage. However, the 6 player is left by themselves to take the powerful line attacks. With the number of posibilities, the 6 player attempts to take the majority of the back court line attacks in this system. Depending on how much of the line is made available for the attacker, the defensive unit may prefer to leave two defenders covering the line.

When the opponents use a fast combination attack, the middle blocker does not have much chance to form a solid blocking unit with the outside blocker. In this case, the middle blocker will inform the 6 defender of this, and tell them to position themselves in between the two blockers (BM-h). The defender is in the prime position to pick up the fast ball that goes between the seam of blockers. If the attack manages to touch a blocker on the way out, the defender in position 6 is in a good position to save the ball.

All in all, the 6 back defensive system can be quite complex and requires a lot of communication and experience to make the defence work well against a number of attacks. There are many variations to this type of defence and it relies heavily on the formation of the block and the way the opponents can attack as well as their attacking abilities.

6.3.3 Flat Line system.

When the players struggle to move around the court, they will often find themselves in a flat line defensive strategy.

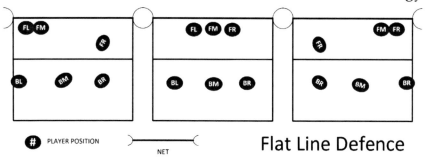

Flat Line Defence

26. Flat Line defence system

This way they cover the court fairly evenly between them. The system is a compromise of the 6-up and 6-back system, where all players can pick up tips, and play over hand defence from long driven balls. They are also in positions to fill the gaps from slow moving blockers, or one-on-one blocking set ups. Typically, all back row players position themselves approximately 2.5-3m from the net and are approximately 2m away from each other.

Players with high ball handling skills can play this system very effectively, as they form a balance on the court, however,

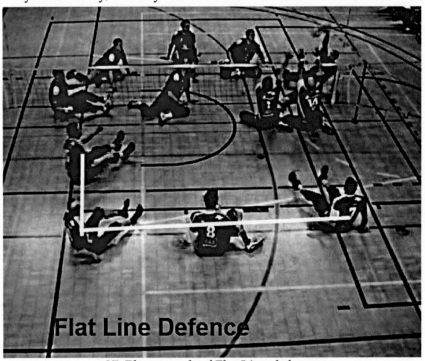

Flat Line Defence

27. Photograph of Flat Line defence

if the team is slow in movement, they have to rely upon a front court setter and two front court attackers, which can make it harder for them to score a point.

Advantages of the flat line defence include;

- Players covering an equal amount of the court at the same time, making it balanced
- Individual utilisation of energies are saved from less movement around the court
- Counter attacks from all parts of the court are possible and at various speeds

Disadvantages of the flat-line defensive system include;

- Players need to have a high level of ball handling to play this effectively

◘ At times, playing the ball is beyond human reaction time capabilities

◘ Counter-attacks can be easier to defend against as there are less front court attackers

The flat-line defence is the most static of defensive systems, but it requires the most amount of skill to play with. When teams cannot always put a double block up in time, the defensive player needs to be in a position to take hard driven spikes to the ground, deep spikes to the edge of the court and tips landing just behind and out of reach of the blocker.

6.4 **Summary**

Choosing a defensive system depends on many variables, such as; amount of training together, the skill sets of the players on your team, the attacking formation, and the strengths of the opponents, amongst others. Often various types of defensive systems need to be trained, while other teams will only operate with one system throughout an entire tournament.

Training players that are used to playing standing volleyball poses issues for sitting volleyball coaches. Many of these actions require specialist technical training and a fair amount of practice in being able to defend the court. The angle of decent from the attacker is very different and the reaction time to react to balls is reduced to almost nothing. Positions of hands are important as they guide the player for movement and for playing the ball. If players have legs and feet, they also play an important role in the keeping the ball off the floor.

SECTION 3
Development in Sitting Volleyball

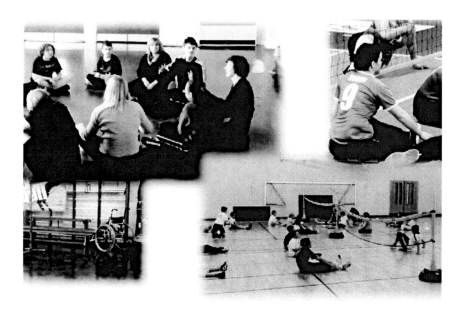

7 YOUTH DISABILITY ISSUES

Before getting into details about how Sitting Volleyball can be used in schools, youth and developmental sports, a brief introduction into terminology is presented. This is being presented in an attempt to avoid misunderstanding between readers of this chapter. In recent years there has been some attention on the politically correct way to frame and describe sub-population groups without offending or creating labels on them that do not fit. An example of this is the way the United Nations changed the *'Convention on the rights of disabled people'* to its current title, the *'Convention on the rights of persons with disabilities'*. This was made in attempt to be on the side of the debate that surrounds placing the emphasis of describing people by the person-first approach and not their demographic group. As such, many suggestions imply that the labelling of *'disabled person'* is a negative thing, it has derogatory connotations, or is it just wrong, and required revision or an assumption that the writer/speaker is ignorant of the disability issues.

While writing in this book, there is no intent to insult people by avoiding the consideration that, when talking about people, it is the person that comes first and not their disability. However there are equally strong arguments that inform the reader, it is acceptable to use phrases such as *'disabled athlete'*, *'disability sports'*, *'disabled children'*, etc., as explained in the preface of the book (see page xv-xvi).

In terms of youth disability sports, much of the development took place since the 1970s. A lot of enthusiasm was placed on training teachers how best to teach children with disabilities. Background knowledge was placed heavily on the perceptions of teachers as teachers with prior experience were experimenting and shared solutions among other teachers. Due to the diverse nature of having disabilities, pedagogy is forever evolving. The didactics in teaching disabled children could be correct in one context, but be harming in another. And as with all subjects, it only takes one bad experience in physical education (PE) to turn the child off from sports for the rest of their life.

PE is different to other curriculum subjects. Its perception can be quite vast as it still isn't mandatory in all countries. Even in some developed countries, PE wasn't a compulsory subject late into the 20th Century. Australia had only adopted PE as part of the 'Health and PE' curriculum in 1989). There are also differences in the approach towards PE. Some countries elect to keep PE separate between the genders while others will encourage as much co-ed activities as possible. PE is also a subject whereby the outcomes of PE are related to social and emotional growth rather than obtaining some specific knowledge like languages, mathematics and science. To achieve this, improvements of motor skills can monitored and that requires pupils to be physically active. As well as improving on this particular physical literacy component, there are other facets that are taught and practice in PE. A large component is motivation and it is largely the responsibility of the teacher to spark a level of motivation for children to be physically active. However, teachers often face difficulties in trying to understand children with disabilities when providing a suitable motivation climate.

The focus of providing teaching material to increase motivation is often based on research however, there are currently very few studies that have investigated disabled children in school sports. Relying on such research could be detrimental to the future of youth disability sports and a deeper understanding of sports from the perspective of disabled children is needed. There seems to be many reasons for the lack of available material from disabled children, which include; difficulties with collecting data; complications in finding valid instruments; vast ranges of disabilities of individuals and; participation consent being withheld.

Of the available findings, much is based on teachers' perception on mainstreaming and has since indicated six areas of focus; support; effects on peers without disabilities; attitudes and intentions of children without disabilities; social interactions; Academic Learning Time in PE of students with disabilities; and training and attitudes of general PE teachers. In terms of how training general PE teachers takes place, the limited studies from youth perspectives have indicated the need for the child to develop a thick skin; making the PE setting a self-affirming environment; making PE a place for pupils to initiate social interaction; and avoiding self-threatening comments about their own sense of self through displaying a happy disposition when in public. All these factors must be recognised when dealing with youth disability sports.

7.1 Schools development

Throughout developed countries in the world, it is a well-known fact that the school time is the only time in a person's life when it is assured they will be physically active. Within the school environment, pupils are graded for PE through assessment of; motor skill competence in various forms; how they actively participate in PE and with others; being knowledgeable of the benefits from physical activity throughout the lifespan; and what they know about the principles of health-related fitness activities.

Although play time, free time and extra curriculum activities stimulate a child's learning, the PE lesson is one where the pupil has a teacher supervising the learning, facilitating achievement through outcomes,. The teachers are professionally trained to deliver these areas. This is not to say that a child without a teacher will not learn motor skills by themselves, but given the social constructs needed for a child's development, the school lesson provides adequate opportunities.

The educator has multiple tasks that aid the child's development. When they are in an environment with children of some disability, they usually find themselves adapting the lesson to suit the needs of the child whilst keeping the other 20 to 30 children occupied. Such methods has come from a movement of inclusion sports which was popularised from the 1970s. Much has happened since in those societies, where the term 'inclusion' was once seen as being equal to dumping disabled children into typical schools settings and that was seen as enough. It was otherwise known as mainstreaming.

Disability sport has been seen as an effective avenue for developing confidence and enhancing friendships, especially for females. In the school environment, a developing child needs an individual educational plan (IEP) to support them throughout school life. This plan involves the child's family, paediatrician and the school. The guidelines in today's educational systems need to adapt to the environment of the child, and specialists should acquire seven competencies; planning; assessment; prescription; teaching /counselling / coaching; evaluation; co-ordination of resources; and lastly, advocacy. This is known in the profession as PAP-TE-CA. The educator would use these competencies when designing an IEP. By following this process, teachers have a mechanism to overcome problems with the development in the child's ecology. As a result, educators find other factors that have an effect on the long-term outcomes of physical activity and sport for youth.

An international call for prioritising inclusive education was made in 1994. The UNESCO Salamanca Statement was signed, and since then many places have increased the number of inclusive schooling environments. Teachers were asked what the top two main aims of inclusion are, and has been well reported that it is to benefit children by increasing their self-perception and social competencies. Particularly, when the disabled child increases his/her confidence, the non-disabled child increases awareness and experiences with people with disabilities and the teacher incorporates creative strategies into their teaching practices. This makes for a modern approach to society.

For the role of inclusion to work, teachers also play a part in realising a philosophy. One such method is to work with unspecialised teachers to share skill learning. With skill sharing taking place, inclusion also highlights the importance to share resources as well as the pupils.

There are three key points to an inclusion philosophy; pupils are treated individually through individualised educational plans; using two systems is costly and illogical as two types of teachers (one for non-disabled, one for disabled) are conducting virtually the same task, when only one is needed; and, segregation of pupils leads to demoralising attitudes, in particular when they are involved in a physical education setting. The three key points presented in the context of physical education relates to the second article of the Salamanca Statement, which states;

> *Regular schools with inclusive orientation are the most effective means of combating discrimination, creating welcoming communities, building an inclusive society and achieving education for all (United Nations Educational, Scientific and Cultural Organisation, 1994, Art.2.)*

In many of the Central and Eastern European countries, the majority of societies believe segregation is better for the child than integration. This could be attributed to the stigma factor associated with families who have a disabled child. Schools seemed to have low resources to include disabled children and doubted if inclusion works. There was a fear that both disabled and non-disabled children would fall back on their academic progress. In accordance with the Salamanca Agreement, some of these countries have placed special schools next to mainstream schools so there is a greater chance of interaction between pupils, although these schools still have separate resources centred at special schools. This has been viewed as a bridge to inclusion. Some other countries, for example, Hungary, were even reluctant to make this first step where stigma against disabilities seems evidently high.

Training programs for people working with disabilities are also quite vast; off the shelf resources by the WHO; British Paralympic Association's Ability vs Ability programme; as well as the Hellenic Paralympic Association's Paralympic Schools' programme were well established in their respective locations. Typically most national federations like, the Finnish Disability Sports Organisations have their own resource cards for pan-disability sport ideas and the Finnish Paralympic Committee have an interactive Paralympic sports booklet. Despite what seems to be a mass of resources for disability sports, Sitting Volleyball material remains thin, unclear and scattered in comparison to other Paralympic sports.

7.2 Disability Models for Sport

There are many types of disabilities, ranging from physical impairments through to intellectual disabilities. Impairment was considered as *"any loss of psychological, physiological or anatomical structure or function"*. To use the term *'disability'* in everyday contexts, there are three common models; the medical model, the social minority model, and the ecological model. In 2001, the World Health Organization modified its definition of disability to include medical, social and ecological models. The medical model, is sometimes referred to as the individual model, is based upon defectiveness and is generally used negatively towards the disabled person. The social model is based on the social differences created that make a person disabled, which in turn began a trend to use the person-first orientation. The ecological model uses the social model and places the environment around the person which is faced on a regular basis. The environment can be defined as having two functions, either barriers or enablers. At the time of writing, this latter theory has seen most amount of societal acceptance and brought changes in the law through a rights-based model.

More recently, an advancement of disability awareness in societies has seen over 150 nations signing up to the United Nations agreement on the Convention on the Rights of Persons with Disabilities (CRPD) and creating a newer, Human Rights Model of disability. Article 30 of the CRPD is titled, 'Participation in cultural life, recreation, leisure and sport' and states;

> *5. With a view to enabling persons with disabilities to partic-ipate on an equal basis with others in recreational, leisure and sporting activities, States Parties shall take appropriate measures:*
>
> *To encourage and promote the participation, to the fullest extent possible, of persons with disabilities in mainstream sporting activities at all levels;*
>
> *To ensure that persons with disabilities have an opportunity to organize, develop and participate in disability-specific sporting and recreational activities and, to this end, encour-age the provision, on an equal basis with others, of appropriate instruction, training and resources;*
>
> *To ensure that persons with disabilities have access to sporting, recreational and tourism venues;*
>
> *To ensure that children with disabilities have equal access with other children to participat[e]ion in play, recreation and leisure and sporting activities, including those activities in the school system;(taken from UN CRPD, 2008, [own emphasis])*

The application of this convention has recently prompted an approach with the term of 'Rights-based model' of disa-bility. This is a current model consisting of strong advocacy towards the human rights of disabled people. To illustrate the differences between the models, a person is describing a young woman using a wheelchair;

> *Medical Model: Oh this poor woman, she should go to a doctor and discuss with him if there is a therapy which could enable her to walk again, like everybody else.*

> *Social Model: The community really should build ramps in front of public buildings, so that persons like her can participate in social life:*
> *Rights-based Model: When she gets a job, her employer will have to build accessible rooms. This is her right! (taken from Heumann, 2008)*

Another area of concern for youth disability sports is the majority of literature in disability studies is based on working aged adults with disabilities. This has led disability research into some problems. The appropriateness of classifying people has only been subjected to the views and experiences of adults. Rather than looking at the individuals throughout their lifespan, it has restricted science's interpretation of youth and disability. Understanding the life of a disabled child could be greatly enhanced if there is more research that helps classify childhood disabilities. It is therefore no surprise that the majority of PE teachers and coaches have low sense of self-efficacy when it comes to working in an inclusion setting. It is also not surprising to encourage disabled children to be physically active as there are more and bigger barriers to physical activity than facilitative enablers. These issues should really be raised and addressed as the future of elite disability sports depends a lot on the youth disability sports issues.

7.3 Disability Sport Issues

What often separates sports like Sitting Volleyball and volleyball is the concept of disability. There are considerations in disabled sport that often get overlooked which are not equated in non-disabled sports. This section looks at some areas that have an effect on inclusive-efficacy values. Issues addressed include the media and significant others. In addition to these two areas of focus, other issues that warrant consideration for disability sports and inclusive-efficacy are not included in this edition. Transportation, costs, sponsorship, competition frameworkds all play an independent role in disability sports.

More information about this can be found from existing literature in disability sports.

7.3.1 **Media.**

The implications of having low media coverage on disability sports can make it difficult for teachers and coaches to find role models. Media also struggles to express clearly the issues of disability sport classification. Inclusive-efficacy remains low until there is accessibility to disability sport in the media, being knowledgeable of sports classification, have been classified, or know someone close enough that has gone through the classification process.

Disability sports are often traced back to the birth of the Paralympics when it was then known as the International Stoke Mandeville Games. Only a few clips of media coverage of these games can be found in the archives, and often media did not show live events. Paralympic coverage remained very low when compared to the Olympic Games. Broadcasters have indicated that the complications of understanding classifications are a drawback for them to show disability as a spectacle. The public mentioned confusion when athletes breaking a world record did not win the event. Since then, Paralympic education programs and information became more accessible through the internet and subscription broadcasting networks. Live broadcasting is programmed into future schedules. The use of stored online videos through the official paralympic channels remain a good source for teachers to see how a sport is played at the top level.

Teachers who do not have access to go to a Sitting Volleyball match, by watching Paralympic Sitting Volleyball on the internet channels will be a good source of increasing their inclusive-efficacy. This can then be shared with the pupils. It is a major source of knowledge as they realise the game is actually played while sitting on the floor. They will get to see how active the sport is. It is also an affordable activity whereby people with a variety of functionality can play together. Converting this knowledge is quite challenging and often media has the responsibility to illustrate how the game is adapted from the Paralympic limelight to a school setting.

Social media is playing an important role. Resources for coaches and teachers can be found on the book's website.

7.3.2 **Significant Others.**

The persistence of an individual's decision to continue with sport into adulthood is often influenced by the significant others of that child, such as; teachers, parents and friends. Studies demonstrated people's behaviour improves as they interact more frequently. The behavioural improvements towards disabled people are also evident through contact with others. A reciprocal determinism takes place whereby, the teacher affects society and society enables the teacher to perform their tasks. Therefore, schools play a significant role in the perception of physical activity for the disabled child.

Compared with non-disabled people, there are fewer opportunities to take up sport beyond school time for people with disabilities. Hence there are fewer opportunities for significant others to engage disabled people into sport. Individuals often feel they have inadequate experiences to deal with the variety of disabilities. Consequently, those uncertainties have been seen to attach stigma through fear to teachers attitudes towards working with disabled people. Training teachers and coaches is a resourceful way to help them overcome such fears. In places where the ethics of teaching is constantly under scrutiny, inclusive training is offered as part of pre-service training (i.e. Teacher degrees) and in-service training or professional development. Even though courses are designed to give knowledge to the teachers, the practicalities of putting the knowledge into practice can often be a daunting one. The same feelings are often found in novice coaches as the instructor is apprehensive of what is and isn't possible to do.

Changing the attitudes of teachers has occasionally been productive, but studies have shown an increase in acquiring the correct attitudes, as low predictors of intentions or actions when promoting physical activities for the disabled. In these cases, teachers reported better attitudes towards inclusive education, but during observations of their class actions, the teachers did not apply inclusion techniques. Perhaps these studies did not allow sufficient time to allow the teachers to make the inclusive environment effective.

7.4 Inclusion Sport

The term inclusion can be used in different ways. At times it can mean social inclusion, whereby there are community programs that facilitate activities for people who are considered to be deprived, ethnic minority, or poorly educated. Often, the programme aims are to provide opportunities for the target groups with the intention to allow them to do the same things as what everyone else is doing, or have experiences and attempts to understand the habits of what people do. These goals can be similar to what inclusion sports can be when they are designed for people with disabilities.

Although social inclusion programs and inclusion sports programs may have related goals, they can be very different programs, and often have been misunderstood by community organisations. Inclusion sports programs are a recognised term in physical education and sport as way for people with and without disabilities to be participating in sports together. It is another step forward from the progress made from integrated sport. Integrated sports once were designed to adapt a sport so that a disabled person could play a sport. In other words, a sport is played in a way whereby people with disabilities would play the game under special circumstances. Often this special treatment has been confused with the need of assistance to perform, that belittles the ability of disabled people to a level of incompetence. In these cases, it is integrated person that is actually doing the activity, but their assistant. Inclusion sports are different because it is a philosophy whereby sports and physical activities exists, where people with and without disabilities participate together and each individual's needs are met.

In this way, Sitting Volleyball has been seen as an inclusive sport. It has been seen as having more inclusion capabilities than most other sports. When teacher trainees were asked to review which of the popular disability sports they thought had the greatest potential for inclusion sports, Sitting Volleyball was ranked highest. Swimming was second and Goalball was third. It should be noted, that these results were based on teacher trainees, in other words, student teachers, and had taken a course in disability sports. Some of them may have lacked experience with teaching. Some experienced teachers were asked the same question after attending some Sitting Volleyball in-service teacher training. They also held the same perception that Sitting Volleyball has the potential to be one of the most inclusive sports. Coaches that have attended short courses in Sitting Volleyball reported an increased awareness of inclusion although the training lacked the possibility to train disabled athletes.

7.4.1 **Range of (Dis)abilities**

In the book, *Teaching Disability sport; a guide for physical educators*, by Ronald Davis, there is a table for types of activities depending on the level of function an individual has. Davis suggests breaking down volleyball into four skills; passing (as in, the underarm and overhand pass), attack-hit, serving, and blocking. Each skill has its own calibrated category based on the level of function of an individual.

Low functional skill levels have been defined as people with *"multiple impairments; unable to sit independently without trunk support; unable to move independently on the floor; might use an electric or power wheelchair".* People with moderate functional skills are defined as, *"Able to sit independently for short durations; can sit independently by bracing with one arm to the floor; has moderate strength in upper body and can momentarily lift buttocks from floor while seated using two arms; able to move 3ft(1m) independently on the floor".* High functionality is defined as, *"Able to sustain a seated position on the floor without support; can lift buttocks from the floor and move 3-6ft (1-1.8m) independently; is able to hold both arms overhead and maintain balance while in seated position without support; is able to lean backward to reach or strike a volleyball without losing balance when seated on the floor".*

Davis then produced a useful chart for teachers and coaches to use for session planning based on the individual skills. This table has been presented in table 2.

Table 2. General modifications for Sitting Volleyball (Reprinted, with permission, from R.W. Davis, 2011. Teaching disability sport: A guide for physical educators (Champaign, IL: Human Kinetics), 126)

Skill level	Skill	Activity modifications
Low	Passing	Roll a ball back and forth across the length of a table to a partner
	Attack	Strike a swinging lightweight ball to simulate an attack-hit
	Block	From 2ft (0.6m) in front of a tabletop, move the wheelchair to block a ball before it rolls off the table's edge. Balls come from any direction.
	Serve	Seated in front of a table with a ball tethered overhead, swing the ball forward over the table to the opposite end to simulate a serve.
Moderate	Passing	Seated on the floor, roll or toss a ball to another student.
	Attack	Seated on the floor beside a tall traffic cone, balance a volleyball on the cone and strike the ball from the cone.
	Block	Seated on the floor beneath a ball tethered to a basketball rim, block the ball with two arms as it swings forward.
	Serve	Throw the ball from a serving position on the floor.
High	All skills	No modifications: used with highest-functioning students.

7.4.2 Mixed Genders

The difference in net height between men and women Sitting Volleyball is 10 centimetres. Up until 1992, teams with women were allowed to compete as mixed teams. A year later, the first women specific tournament was the European championships in Järvenpää, Finland. Nowadays, top tournaments will only be separated, although very often, women will compete with men in mixed club teams. In some leagues, these leagues will have a net that is set at 1.10m and others will force women to play at the height of a men's net (1.15m).

Some youth national teams also feature female players as a way for giving exposure to elite competition. In these tournaments, the net is at 1.15m. Sitting Volleyball demonstrates again the flexibility it has towards the inclusion of different people with various abilities to play with each other.

7.4.3 Obesity

In recent times, there has been a lot of attention on obesity and the need to be physically active. People that are clinically obese are in danger of becoming disabled. The use of devices to help them with their mobility is become more and more widespread. Public spaces once exclusive for people with disabilities are being occupied by people confronted with obesity. A person morphs from normal weight to overweight and obese usually involves a combination of over eating of poor quality food and insufficient exercise. Which makes it hard to motivate individuals to take up exercise. Sitting Volleyball may serve to be an alternative to this problem.

The amount of exercise an individual does during the day should contribute to the overall minimum recommended amount of daily exercise. Large amount of evidence is produced to show that a lack of exercise is more harmful than smoking. People who are smokers and are physically active live longer than those who do not smoke and do not exercise. Furthermore, even doing half the recommended amounts of physical activity will increase the average lifespan of an individual. There are many interested groups looking to change sedentary behaviours. This can be achieve by making gradual changes. Clear answers on whether low to moderate amount of exercises can combat the obesity epidemic are slowly building momentum. Sitting Volleyball can be seen as an activity that fulfils low, moderate and vigorous physical activity levels. It could also prompt a newer set of guidelines from 60 minutes of moderate to vigorous physical activities levels per day, five times a week, to indicate the total duration of low to moderate physical activity levels that are needed to remain healthy.

It is likely that Sitting Volleyball can be suitable activity for this target group. There are social as well as skill and personality factors that would benefit from a challenging game like Sitting Volleyball. The risks from participating in sports for people with obesity are reduced as running can cause joint impact and falling from breathlessness is minimised. Movement can be acute hence allowing for regulated exercise. After working out, people are encouraged to shower and maintain good hygiene.

7.5 Summary of Youth Disability Issues

The issue of youth and disability is forever expanding. In addition to the lack of knowledge in this particular area of interest, there are growing numbers of children with reported disabilities or long-term illnesses. There are widely known benefits from exercising that include physical and mental well-being of individuals. This should be the same for children too, and in particular children with disabilities. However, disabled children often find it hard to find activities to be regularly physically active, due to a number of social and environmental factors. Recent attention towards the rights of children with disabilities is a process that will take time. In the meantime training of teachers and coaches can start to embrace the inclusion philosophies.

As children live in a fast paced world, there are two main sources where adolescents are fed information outside of school. The media plays an important part in educating and raising awareness of disability sports. In addition to enabling children into sport, the media can provide role models that children can aspire to be like. Friends become more significantly involved into the decision making of the growing youth. Family involvement and support is forever essential, but it could be said that the main purpose for schooling is to prepare the child for adult life. Hence, being part of society is important and having a good social network and the rights to socialisation can enhance physical activity levels.

7.5.1 Further readings

Block, M. (2007). *A Teacher's Guide to Including Students with Disabilities in General Physical Education, 3rd. Edition.* Paul H. Brookes Publishers

Brittain, I. (2009). *The Paralympic Games Explained.* Routledge

Davis, R. (2011). *Teaching Disability sport; a guide for physical educators.* Human Kinetics

DePauw, K. & Gavron, S. (2005). *Disability and Sports. 2nd Edition.* Human Kinetics

Fitzgerald, (2009). *Youth Disability Sports.* Routledge

Gilbert, K. & Schanz, O. (2009). *The Paralympic Games: Empowerment Or Sideshow?* Meyer & Meyer

Horvat, M., Block, M. & Kelly, L. (2007). *Developmental and adapted physical activity assessment.* Human Kinetics

Heumann, J. (2008). *Disability in Action.*

Sherrill, C. (2004). *Adapted physical activity, recreation, and sport: cross-disciplinary and lifespan. 6th Edition.* McGraw-Hill

Thurmeier, R., Gustafson, P. & Goodwin, D. (2004). Reactions to the Metaphors of Disability: The Mediating Effects of Physical Activity. *Adapted physical Activity Quaterly,* 21(4). 379-398

The Salamanca Statement and Framework

UN Enable – UN CRPD

8 JUNIOR COMPETITIONS

The launch of long term athletic development models since the middle of the 1990s have seen a rise in the number of small sided games for youth sports. Part of the long term athletic development model by Istvan Balyi it is to enable young people with the opportunity to play sport, by improving their fundamentals. Its purpose is to enhance participation and performance in sport. In the model, there are 6 stages; 1. *FUNdamentals* (5-7years); 2. *Learning to Train* (7-11years); 3. *Training to Train* (12-15years); 4. *Training to Compete* (16-19years); 5. *Training to Win* (20-23 years); and, 6. *Retaining* (24years and up). The recommended ages can have 2 years discrepancy in each direction. For each stage, there are key performance components, including; endurance; strength; flexibility; speed; and, skills. Also, according to philosophies in the development of children, chronological age plays a role in each stage. Along with chronological age, there is training age and biological age. Training age is defined by the amount of time the child has been sports training, and biological age relates to growth spurts and body maturity.

With the key performance components, children will often go through neuropsychological development stages. The most often used way of approach is based on Jean Piaget stages of cognitive development, and has the following 4 stages;

Sensorimotor (birth-2years); *Preoperational* (2-7years); *Concrete operational* (7-11years); and, *Formal operational* (11years and up). Hence, the majority of youth sports competition models uses the concrete operational – learning to train phase and the formal operational – training to train stages.

People with disabilities may sometimes be lagging behind the average stage that their peers are at, whether it is from the cognitive development or athletic models. As such, guidelines for youth disability sports competitions may be a little more complicated. There are many principles for inclusion, and there are many formats. They all have their own merits and their own faults, and this is what makes it very difficult for teams to engage in competition, as structure is not uniform between various schools of thoughts.

Specially adapted fitness tests are available for the phys-ically disabled. There are also popular motor tests that have been used across the globe as a form of battery testing. The Bruininks-Oseretsky test of motor proficiency-2 has 8 relevant components for Sitting Volleyball. Tests are grouped in the simple adaptable ways, as represented in table 3;

Table 3. Bruininks-Oseretsky Test of Motor Proficiency-2 Adaptations for Sitting Volleyball

Component	Adaptation
Bilateral Co-ordination	Catch and Throw
Upper limb Co-ordination	Clapping, Finger connections
Running speed and agility	Floor shuffling from A to B
Upper limb speed and dexterity	Arms go Left, Right, Front, and Up
Balance	Push ball against wall Pull ball against someone
Strength	Forward overhead throw of ball (Throw –in) Backward over arm throw of ball.
Response speed	Test under command to move left or right, and deduct time from original speed test
Visual motor control	Reading Ball flight, Clap on peak and bounce.

Volleyball testing of children game levels can be modified to the sitting court with similar outcomes. Results from tests from Helmen, Brady, or Allen are tried and tested ways of testing volleyball skill abilities. Other types of test that might be useful to conduct include psychomotor tests such as; Body attitude test; Body shape questionnaire; Rosenburg Self-Esteem scale; Harter's Self-Perception Instruments; and, Self-Description questionnaires.

Combining results from other activities may also be relevant for creating adapted games for Sitting Volleyball. Making recommendations based on an IEP can be time consuming and the knowledge base might be limited to offer an effective programme. Nonetheless, outlines for youth competitions are generally encouraged by many.

8.1 Small sided games

The long term athletic development model has increased the number of possibilities to develop small sided games. The term small sided games, is defined by having less team members in the team sports and games have modifications from the full adult game. For Sitting Volleyball, it is essentially a team sport hence the reduction of team members can be reduced to one-a-side through to six-a-side on a smaller court. Sitting Volleyball is a game based on the adaptations of indoor standing volleyball, whereby the court is smaller, and the net is lower, so it could be feasible to say that it is a small sided game of volleyball. It is also possible for physical educators to avoid changing anything else to the game and plan using Sitting Volleyball. Alternatively, teachers may make further modifications to smaller sided games with ease.

Based on the mini-volley models of volleyball for youth, mini-Sitting Volleyball could also be introduced. There are very limited resources to guide on how to do this, and this could be a reason for the low amounts of youth participation in Sitting Volleyball. There are probably a lot of others as well, but according to much research in physical education, youth sports and inclusion of youth in physical activities, if there is no knowledge of the game for youth, then it is virtually impossible for youth to consciously play the game.

Small sided games have the advantages of;

- Increased active participants
- Increased contact with the ball
- Increased skill development
- Increased opportunities to play cooperative games
- Increased opportunities to play competitive games

By making minor adaptations to youth volleyball programs around the world, the prospect of children as young as 6 years old through to adult age is hereby available. Although the modifications to the games can be further adapted, to suit the children, the following information can be useful to use as a flexible template.

8.1.1 6-8 year olds

At this age, many children will find themselves exploring the fundamentals of movement. Children need careful facilitation of movement skills covering internal and external control. Balance, coordination and agility are main components in a "fundamentals of movement" program. Based on basic movements which are necessarily for skill development, children will need to learn to adjust their own movements to the ball flight phenomenon. For children learning this, the 2 dimensions of movement is a critical path for these young children. Mastering 2D will lead to greater chances of success in ball sports. This later becomes 3 dimensional movements, whereby width and length is combined with height of the ball flight.

As children are learning a lot and gaining a lot of stimuli at the same time, it could be said that children need to be playing individually in order to acquire sufficient amounts of skill to play the sport later on. Although skill development is crucial at this age, game play is just as important to incorporate into a fun learning programme. Games based on one a side would therefore encourage the use of the skills necessary in recognising ball flight and the challenges of beating an opponent. As children learn to use their new movement skills based on sitting on the floor, they can explore best ways to cover the court and improving reaction time to play the ball.

Suitable competition measures of 1.5m x 1.5m give the child room to play the game like short tennis, as well as controlling the ball for while setting up their own attacks. Many concepts of learning can be fitted into this game. A low net will increase the rate of play, although 90cm is a reasonable height that is a suitable challenge for them to play. To encourage more rallies, the net can be raised higher. If the players want more encouragement to score more points, then a larger court space can be made. Courts that are too big for the player to cover will reduce the amount of encouragement in playing, and then could be detrimental to overall development of the player. Finding the right court sizes is not rocket science, but can be treated as an opportunity for children to discover their range of movements.

8.1.2 **9-11 year olds**

The introduction of another player into the game per side commences the beginning of team sports for these young children. By playing as a team, a lot of the decision making takes place. Players learn more than just the acute skill to move and play by acquiring decision making and communication skills between team mates. At this age, children are placed into pairs so they can play with each other. Reinforcement of the rules to play the ball among the team members before sending the ball over the net will enhance the outcomes of individual development.

By playing in pairs, the dynamics of team play are introduced, and high levels of involvement in game play are continually available for the team mates. Introduction of skills such as the serve and underhand pass are core components of the child development at this age. Players will start to decide who will take the ball and how they will share the space between them. To enable this, players are encouraged to play on a court that is 3m wide. As part of the space sharing experience, a court that is 4m long will help children of this age to move forward and backwards as they play the ball, as well as develop greater awareness of tactics in how to play.

8.1.3 **12-13 years old**

As children enter a formal operational age, they acquire more solution based outcomes. The introduction of a third team member helps the players learn to use attack and defensive tactics without over complicating the development of skills. 3 a side games are useful for youth development as systems built on 3 a side are often segments of the 6 a side game.

The width of the court is covered by three players, but often one of the players will act as the team setter. As such, 3.5m width was recommended. A total length of 6m will encourage teams to transition from defence to offense. The teams can start thinking about how to play, and how best to cover the court between them. Using the maximum of three touches between the players can also encourage each player to have a role of touching the ball before the ball is sent over the net. A lot of emphasis on team play can be generated at this level of game play. Key aspects to build the attack are the spike and block. The spike can become a useful shot to develop, and with the spike, the block can also be learnt too.

Teams may find it is better for them to stay away from the net. In this way, they play in a system similar to a flat line defensive system. This system encourages a lot of forward movement of the player from the right of the court. It also mimics the backrow setting from position 1. If the player on the right has to play the first ball, then the player on the left can move forward to set the ball. In the meantime, the middle player can either act as back middle player, fast middle player, or can try to swing outside to attack the ball from where the setter had come from (in the first case, attack the ball from the right, in the second case, attack the ball from the left). Trying to play this system demands a lot of understanding of volleyball components, such as space, timing, environment, and people.

8.1.4 **14 years old**

This is the last age group of children whereby they play the game that is not 6 a side. This next progression is four a side volleyball. A lot of emphasis on tactics is obtained through playing this game. Previously, formal operational phases were solution based, now they are starting to generate hypotheses. Children biological age is old enough to start using free weights and gain extra strength. The transition from defence to offence is used a lot during rallies. The movement from front court blocking to back court defending back to front court offense is used frequently at this level, and reinforces the required states in the 6 a side game.

There are two main ways of playing the four a side game, the diamond shape, where the setter stays at the net in the middle of the court, and there is also the two up and two back systems. Both are effective ways of playing. If the players can play the ball behind them, otherwise known as a reverse set, they might be able to play the diamond system. The simplest system is to use the 2up and 2 back offensive system as it keeps the players directed to play the ball to the setter who would be at the front right side of the court, and the attacker players the ball from the front left side of the court.

A separation between the front and back zones is also introduced. Since the full game only permits 3 players at any one time to be in the front zone, a zone that separates the front and back court players is needed. The rules become much more complex than in previous small sided games. The player who serves is not allowed to play in the front zone. The team work that gets built up from this game is more like the full game as there will be periods of rallies that some players have an active role, but do not actually contact the ball.

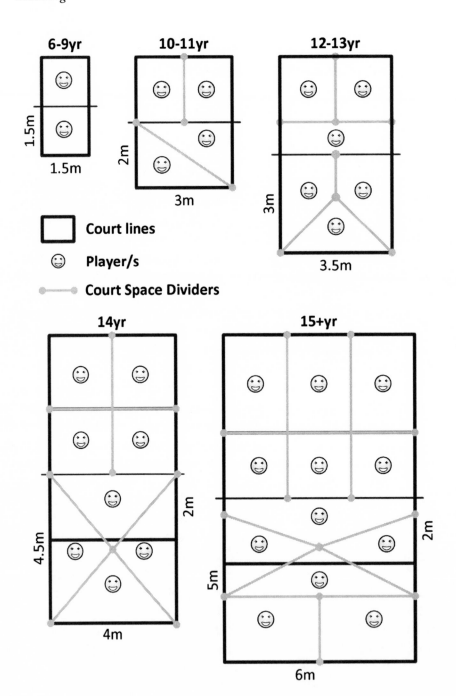

28. Recommended Small Sided Court Dimensions

8.1.5 **15+ years old**

At this age, youth are encouraged to play the full adult game. Although players may not be fully grown, the net height for boys and girls should remain the same as women's height (1.05m). Only when boys are playing after the age of 17, should the net be move up to full men's height net (1.15m).

Players will find that their abilities to play are completed, with the introduction of libero players and a variety of attacking options. A full size court can also be played on so that players learn to move and play with efficiency. If the players start to show certain characteristics, they might want to start learning the role of a specialist player. Perhaps they are better at setting than attacking, or they might be good at blocking but poor at reception.

Children are developing themselves, and it might be too early to put too much effort into specialising the player's skills. There are some well stated arguments against doing so. Training must emphasis on all round development of the individual. The teacher or coach might have the challenge the balance of learning and improving, compared to frustration of doing something over and over without much success. The individual may prefer to work on their strengths. As the child develops and limb lengths change, a highly supportive environment is often needed to keep the motivation up against the distractions that adolescents often face at this age.

Table 4. Summary of Developmental Stages

Age	Court	Net	Team	Skills
6-9	1.5 x 3m	0.90m	1v1	Catch, throw, volley
9-11	3 x 4m	0.95m	2v2	Underarm pass, service
12-13	3.5 x 6m	1.00m	3v3	Attack, block
14	4m x 9m (2m)	1.05m	4v4	Overarm service, Reverse Setting
15+	6m x 10m (2m)	1.05m	6v6	Specialist roles

8.2 **Intellectual Disabilities**

Game progression for children with intellectual disabilities requires quite a different approach to the traditional athletic development models. This is partly because children with these types of disabilities have a different way of development. The diversity in the range of disabilities is also vast, and sometimes there are behavioural problems too.

Activities often involve carers as facilitators and the role of inclusion sports plays a prominent part. Reactions might be slow and the sensitivity to surfaces could be great. Further adaptations to the rules might include net height, number of players, the number of contacts permitted, and the types of shots played.

One version of the game is to encourage the movement of player in a circular movement around the court when the ball has been sent over the net. This promotes a lot of movement and excitement. Another way is to fix the centre point of the court, and the player must move to the centre of the court after they play the ball over the net. Common games that involve relay races can help energise a session. However overuse of this method needs to be monitored. When teams have to pass the ball to each other the fastest can encourage focus on team work, skill and communication. Target games provide a goal for the individuals that make volleyball flexible, fun and measurable. Probably the most complex adaptation is a game that encourages the ability to teach space sharing. The goal of this game is to illustrate sharing the court with other people through fun games. Using a variety of balls and the help of assistances to feed the ball to the child can help accelerate the learning.

Whichever way the game might be modified, the various ways to get the game going as well as enhance physical activity is often determined by the abilities of the learner, facilities, and others involved in the class. Children with various disabilities that include intellectual may find that they have high supportive needs. It may take a long time for the child to be able to volley a ball and this may mean the child is static on the floor. Therefore, a separation of skills would be useful before incorporating both movement and skill. The nature of the game may no longer be challenging for others as much as it is for a player who struggles to volley the ball. In this case, differentiation is often advised among physical educators so that each child has the opportunity and right to physical activity.

Due to so many differences between children with intellectual disabilities and a shortage of space to include in this book, no further information is presented here. This is in recognition for the need on more publications as teacher and coach guides of volleyball for intellectual disabilities. Although Sitting Volleyball at the most competitive level is a sport that is played by those with physical disabilities, and not by those with intellectual disabilities, it does not necessarily mean that volleyball cannot be played by intellectual disabilities. Volleyball does appear in the Special Olympics programme as a competition team game as well as an individual skill activity. Sitting Volleyball however does not feature in such programmes. Sitting Volleyball can be seen as a demanding sport, but it could be said that it isn't as demanding to teach as indoor volleyball. The use of some tests designed to assess individual skills and therefore provide information on improvement levels can be an effective tool for teachers.

8.3 Sitting Volleyball as a learning progression

Sitting Volleyball modifies volleyball as a learning progression. The skills of attacking can be enhanced since the athlete can concentrate on the swing of the arm, instead of concentration on the timing of the jump, which can be a difficult task for people to master. The same could be said about the block. By eliminating the timing of jumping in relation to the skill of blocking, players who are already sat on the floor can coordinate their arms for correct blocking techniques. Young players who have difficulty in controlling their service reception will find practicing while sitting useful. The players learn to anticipate the ball quicker whilst on a Sitting Volleyball court as there is less time for the ball to travel over the net. Players often find that they will use the overhand reception shot while sitting down and learn to control the ball towards the setter. During service, the ball can be served with a fast and flat ball, but to control the weight of the ball so that it lands in the court is more challenging when there is a service block. Such a serve can become effective for indoor volleyball players. In the indoor game, players who jump the highest end up having an advantage over others. A particular instance takes place during the attack and block. Attackers aim to jump higher than the block so that they can hit the ball downwards with force. In Sitting Volleyball, the physical limb length removes the essentials of jumping, and instead improves hitting angles of the attacker. When an attacker is faced with a block, the attacker has to do something to avoid losing a point. Therefore, Sitting Volleyball can help an attacker see the block during attack, as well as adjust the attack shot according to the block.

Therefore there are many ways in which Sitting Volleyball practice and game play can improve skills for volleyball. As well as drills for novice volleyball players, these practices can also be utilised for players with intellectual disabilities.

8.4 Concluding thoughts.

All in all, the game can be played among people with and without disabilities, physical or intellectual. As an inclusive game, people who feel compassionate in playing sports together irrespective of a person's current status will find Sitting Volleyball pleasurable game. As a new game to some, people who find themselves without motivation to exercise and play sports can easily find Sitting Volleyball as a solution to their worries. In this way, the art of coaching or pedagogy that for sitting volleyball can seen as a compassionate way of coaching, very much so whereby peace and friendship instilled among elite athletes can continue on in elite competitions.

The versatility of Sitting Volleyball is ever more apparent with a broader variety of backgrounds and types of players that can play this game together. In this book, a brief history of the game in the most competitive format has been explained as has examples of the use of Sitting Volleyball in schools. For the sport to flourish in physical, technical, tactical, and psychological aspects, more collection of games, advance and clinics is needed.

A suggested junior competition model has been presented. It is up to readers, youth clubs and schools, national federations and other major youth competition organisers to consider how to test and implement the youth development of Sitting Volleyball. A flexible approach that encourages critical analysis and feedback on existing competitions can help develop this inclusive game to reach its potential.

Sitting Volleyball was once played only in Europe has spread fast around the world with regular events that could look attractive on the FIVB Calendar. Future developments of the game may find the need to see a closer relationshiop between the FIVB and WOVD with a view for a long term and single body for all forms of volleyball. Since the first suggestions were made by the IPC that there could be a combined international federation, both the FIVB and WOVD have undergone structural changes, new Presidents and experienced very successful Summer Games. Furthermore, both the International Olympic and Paralympic Committees have started a close working partnership. These are positive signs to make volleyball and sitting volleyball grow more.

Finally, this book as tried to emphasis that Sitting Volleyball is played sitting down. While most people associate sitting down as being sedentary and obedient, Sitting Volleyball can be quite active and it certainty is not resting.

Notes

Notes

Notes